CLIT-OLOGY

MASTER EVERY MOVE FROM A TO G-SPOT TO GIVE HER ULTIMATE PLEASURE

Jordan LaRousse & **Samantha Sade**
Authors of *Mastering Your Man from Head to Head*

© 2011 Quiver
Text © 2011 Jordan LaRousse and Samantha Sade
Photography © 2011 Quiver

First published in the USA in 2011 by
Quiver, a member of
Quayside Publishing Group
100 Cummings Center
Suite 406-L
Beverly, MA 01915-6101
www.quiverbooks.com

The publisher maintains the records relating to images in this book
required by 18 USC 2257. Records are located at Rockport Publishers,
Inc., 100 Cummings Center, Suite 406-L, Beverly, MA 01915-6101.

ISBN: 978-1-59233-486-5

Digital edition published in 2011
eISBN-13: 978-1-61058-165-3

Library of Congress Cataloging-in-Publication Data available

Cover design by Traffic
Book design by Kathie Alexander
Photography by Holly Randall
Illustration by Robert Brandt
Printed and bound in Singapore

To Emmanuelle Morgen—
thank you for being our champion and friend.
We will always be grateful to you for
everything you've done for us.

And always, to Joe.

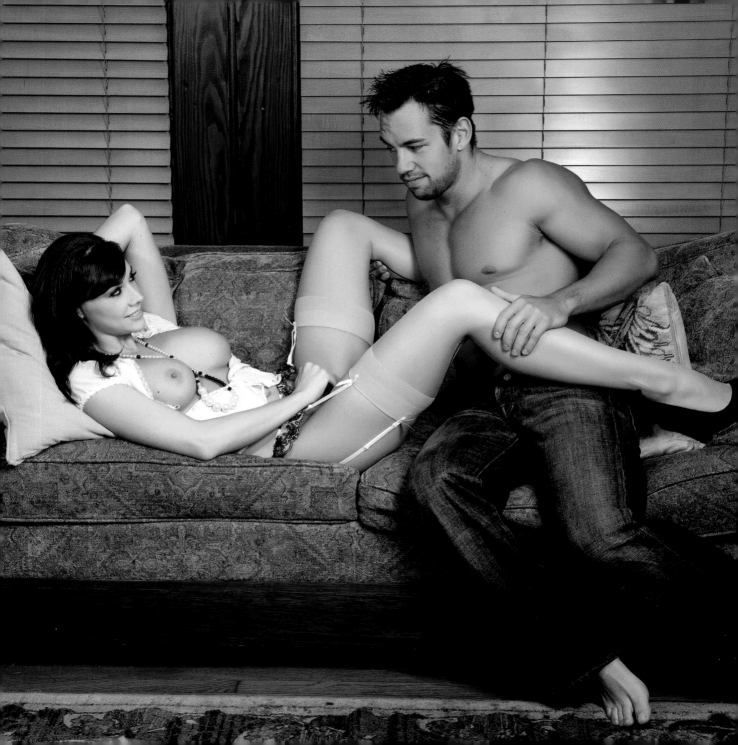

CONTENTS

Why This Is the Must-Read Book for Men Who Want Pussy

Men love pussy. They love it so much that in their lifelong quest to get some, men have gone to great extremes: from writing music to creating impressive works of art to starting fistfights and outright wars—think of Helen of Troy, whose amazing puss launched a thousand ships. Some have even risked everything for it, only to become embroiled in tumultuous sex scandals (yes, we're talking to you Tiger Woods, John Edwards, and Bill Clinton).

But once a man gets some, will he know what to do with it? As loving as a pussy (and the woman attached to it) can be, she can also be a fickle thing if not treated well. Any man who wants to know how to get pussy, and keep on getting it, whether from a tried-and-true partner or from a bevy of babes, needs to read this book. You'll be fully trained on how to coax your pretty kitty out into the open, and how to keep her satisfied and hopping onto your lap, again and again.

Disclaimer

In our effort to turn you into a bona fide clit-ologist, we spent months researching the best information. However, the advice given in this book is meant to be informative and entertaining; it is not meant to take the place of the professional advice of your physician or licensed sex therapist. Also, please be aware that you are fully responsible for anything you do or try in your sex life, so enjoy the tips in this book at your own risk. Be smart, be safe, be responsible, and have fun.

Why We Use Dirty Words

Plain and simple—we love them! There's just nothing like the properly placed dirty word, inside the bedroom or out. But moreover, we use words like *cock, pussy, balls,* and *fuck* because they properly and specifically describe what we're writing about with the beauty of real life. In real life we don't say, "Please insert your penis into my vagina, honey," and we won't write that way, either.

Sources for Clit-ology

The information in this book comes from a variety of resources, including scientific journals, sex manuals (specifically, *The Guide to Getting it On!* by Paul Joannides, *Human Sexuality: Diversity in Contemporary America* by Bryan Strong, *Human Sexual Response* by William H. Masters and Virginia E. Johnson, *The New Good Vibrations Guide to Sex* by Cathy Winks and Anne Semans, and *She Comes First* by Ian Kerner), expert interviews, personal interviews, and two unscientific online surveys.

Clit-ology Surveys

Using an anonymous online sex survey, we gathered intimate information from 420 women and 259 men. Many participants found the survey links at an online magazine for literary erotica, OystersandChocolate.com, so we assume that most, if not all, respondents were at least sexually open enough to read erotic short stories. Many of the colorful quotes, statistics, graphs, and charts in this book are extrapolated from this survey, but please keep in mind that we are not scientists, nor are we professional statisticians. Any identifying information attached to direct quotes, such as names, ages, and occupations, has been altered to protect the anonymity of the speaker.

Expert Sources

JOCELYN HART attended the nurse midwifery program at Columbia University and is a practicing midwife in New York City. In addition to "catching" hundreds of babies and working with pregnant women every day, she has presented at the Babeland store on the topic of sex after childbirth.

JENNI SKYLER, PHD, MS.ED., is a sex therapist and board-certified sexologist. She is the director of the Intimacy Institute for Sex and Relationship Therapy in Boulder, Colorado, and holds a doctorate in clinical sexology and a master's of education in counseling psychology and marriage and family therapy. She writes the column "Sophisticated Sex" for *Boulder Weekly* and "Sexpress Yourself" for *Kraze* magazine.

LAUREN WOLF is the owner of SignatureSensuality.com, a woman-friendly sex toy store. Since 2008, Lauren has been helping to bridge the gap between women and their sensuality. Her bachelor's degree in molecular biology allows Lauren to approach sexuality, sensuality, and intimacy with an interest in both the science and the emotion behind them.

Quiz: Are You a Certified Clit-Ologist?

Do you have what it takes to make your lady happy, horny, hot, and satisfied? Let's find out what *you* know about female sexuality to determine whether you are a true clit-ologist or, if not, just how far you have to go to get your degree.

....

1. What is The Clitoris?

a. A pea-size nub located on the top of her vulva that, when pressed repeatedly, makes her orgasm

b. A sexual organ, composed of eighteen separate parts, that has the sole purpose of bringing her pleasure

c. A sexual organ, composed of four separate parts, that has the sole purpose of bringing her pleasure

d. A pea-size nub located on the top of her vulva that, when caressed and licked, makes her orgasm

e. A medical device that is used to measure the strength and intensity of the female orgasm

2. What and where is the G-spot?

a. Also known as a Guy-spot or Man-cave, it's usually found in the basement or the garage, and it's where your wife or girlfriend sends you when she's annoyed with your antics.

b. It's that little strip of flesh that runs between her pussy and her butthole, otherwise known as the taint.

c. It's a small gland located on her cervix that feels great pleasure when you push your penis in as deep as possible.

d. It's an area of spongy, erectile tissue located on the upper wall of the vagina about 1 to 3 inches (2.5 to 7.6 centimeters) inside.

e. It's a walnut-size gland located about an inch (2.5 centimeters) inside her butthole.

3. When was the first vibrator invented and for what purpose?

a. In the 1880s; it was invented by English Dr. Joseph Mortimer Granville to treat patients suffering from muscle aches.

b. In 1978; it was a handheld device first used on-set by American porn star Marilyn Chambers.

c. In 1994; it was a loud, vibrating prop used by American performance artist Marilyn Manson.

d. In 1987; it was introduced by English sexologist Dr. Eric Cartman as a device intended to treat preorgasmic women (women who have never had an orgasm).

e. In 400 BC during the Yayoi period in ancient Japan; the Japanese courtesans filled a stick of hollow bamboo with small pebbles that "vibrated" when women used them during sex acts.

4. WHAT MALE ATTRIBUTE DO WOMEN RANK HIGHEST IN TERMS OF BEING SEXUALLY ATTRACTIVE?

a. His ability to catch and kill antelope

b. His personality

c. The size of his feet, hands, and penis

d. The angle of his dangle

e. How in shape he is (whether he sports a keg or a six-pack)

5. WHICH STATEMENT IS TRUE ABOUT LUBRICATION AND SEX?

a. Lubrication can be produced by the G-spot.

b. Lubrication is largely produced as a result of increased blood flow to the vagina, which causes the vaginal walls to "sweat."

c. Lubrication can be produced by applying liberal doses of over-the-counter personal lubricant.

d. Lubrication is always a sure sign that she is aroused and ready to go.

e. Both a, b, and c

f. All of the above

6. WHAT IS THE NUMBER ONE RULE FOR GIVING YOUR LADY A SEXY FINGERING EXPERIENCE?

a. Make sure your nails are smooth and trimmed and your hands are clean.

b. Make sure to always wear latex gloves.

c. Make sure to use an antibacterial lubricant, like hand sanitizer.

d. Make sure to only use a maximum of three fingers; otherwise you run the risk of tearing.

e. Both b and c

7. WHAT IS THE BEST WAY TO GIVE A GIRL AN ORGASM?

a. Vigorous thrusting

b. Dirty talk whispered in her ear

c. Spending at least twenty-one minutes on foreplay

d. Buying her expensive jewelry

e. It's one of the great mysteries of the ages.

8. HOW CAN YOU TELL FOR SURE WHETHER YOUR PARTNER IS HAVING AN ORGASM?

a. Her face and chest will turn red.

b. Her labia will darken, and the glans of the clitoris will retract beneath its hood.

c. She will ask for a cigarette.

d. She will use words that would make a sailor blush, and she'll scream like a banshee.

e. Both a and b

9. WHAT IS VAJAZZLING?

a. A sex move wherein you give her mons veneris a raspberry kiss with your tongue and lips

b. The act of tickling her vagina with your finger tips

c. The application of glitter and jewels to the mons veneris where pubic hair used to be

d. The practice of shaving her pubic hair into the shape of a diamond

e. The act of dazzling a woman to have sex with you by giving her jewelry

10. WHAT IS FEMORAL INTERCOURSE?

a. A sexual position named after the Greek goddess Femora in which the woman lies under the man missionary style but props her legs up over his shoulders

b. A two-pronged approach to sex in which the female ("fem") first conducts oral sex to arouse her partner and then immediately transitions to intercourse

c. The scientific term for when a couple is having intercourse solely for the purpose of procreation

d. Rubbing the penis between her thighs, outer labia, and vulva—dry humping without the clothes

e. None of the above

11. WHEN DOES SPLASH CONCEPTION OCCUR?

a. When a couple has unprotected anal sex and the semen drips from her anus into her vagina and impregnates her

b. When the lightbulb suddenly goes off for a guy and he realizes how important clitoral stimulation is for orgasm

c. When a woman comes so much (usually after multiple orgasms), her lover feels like he's splashing around in her juices

d. When a woman surprises her lover with a threesome in the swimming pool

e. It's another term for in vitro fertilization.

12. WHEN A WOMAN EXPERIENCES FEMALE EJACULATION, THE SUBSTANCE THAT SHE "SQUIRTS" IS:

a. Urine. She's just letting loose and peeing on you, dude—it's another term for golden showers.

b. It doesn't really exist. The ejaculate one sees in the porno movies is faked; it's just sugar water expelled by a tiny device called the ejaculizer that the filmmakers keep well hidden.

c. It's a clear, alkaline fluid that originates in paraurethral glands, in the area of the spongy tissue that surrounds the urethra.

d. It's actually semen from the last time you had sex. She's expelling it with her super-fit vaginal muscles.

e. It's a vaginal fluid that comes from the ovaries and through the cervix; squirting usually occurs when she's ovulating.

13. Which statement about female desire and female orgasms is false?

a. If a woman doesn't orgasm during sex with a man, it means that she feels little or no emotional connection with him. Female orgasm is directly linked to emotion.

b. Marilyn Monroe didn't experience orgasms with any of her husbands.

c. When a woman orgasms, her body experiences a release of oxytocin, which makes her feel relaxed and more connected to the person she just had that orgasm with.

d. Certain yoga poses can increase blood flow to the genitals, thereby increasing sexual desire.

e. A woman is more likely to be naturally attracted to your scent if you have a different genetic immune system profile than she does.

14. According to the OystersandChocolate.com survey, the largest number of women are interested in what kinky predilections or fetishes?

a. Foot fetishes

b. Cross-dressing (she wants you to wear her high heels)

c. Swinging (switching partners)

d. BDSM (bondage, domination, submission, and sadomasochism)

e. Water sports (incorporating pee play into sex play)

f. Women aren't really into kink. They'd rather you just pick up your dirty socks off the floor from time to time.

Answer Key

1. b, 2. d, 3. a, 4. b, 5. e, 6. a, 7. c, 8. e, 9. c, 10. d, 11. a, 12. c, 13. a, 14. d

Give yourself one point for each correct answer. If you scored:

0–3 CORRECTLY, you are a clit novice.

4–6 CORRECTLY, you are a clit student.

7–10 CORRECTLY, you are a clit professional.

11–13 CORRECTLY, you are a clit commander.

ALL 14 CORRECTLY, you are a certified clit-ologist. Congratulations!

CHAPTER 1

VulvAnatomy

A Comprehensive Atlas to Your Favorite Lass

The bit of landscape that lies between her legs is complex terrain. From the outer labia to the inner vaginal canal, this chapter gives you a topographical map of the beautiful geography that comprises her vulva, clitoris, and vagina.

If you feel a little lost when gazing into the wonder that resides between your lady's parted legs, don't worry—you're not alone. What's "down there" should be a simple matter of biology, but scientists, experts, and researchers have been scratching their heads over what's what for an absurdly long time. Even today, well into the twenty-first century, they haven't yet figured it all out. The writers of a 2008 college textbook on human sexuality admitted "In spite of what we do know, researchers are finding that we haven't yet mapped all of the basic body parts of women, especially as they relate to the microprocesses of sexual response. Issues like the average size of the clitoris, the existence and function of the G-spot, the role of orgasm and the placement of the many nerves that spider through the pelvic cavity still loom large."[1]

We've taken a look at an array of information and put together what we believe is a useful and comprehensive atlas to your favorite piece of ass. (Don't tell her we said that, though!)

STAN: "HOW DO YOU MAKE A WOMAN LIKE YOU MORE THAN ANY OTHER GUY?"

CHEF: "THAT'S EASY. YOU JUST GOTTA FIND THE CLITORIS."

– SOUTH PARK: BIGGER, LONGER & UNCUT

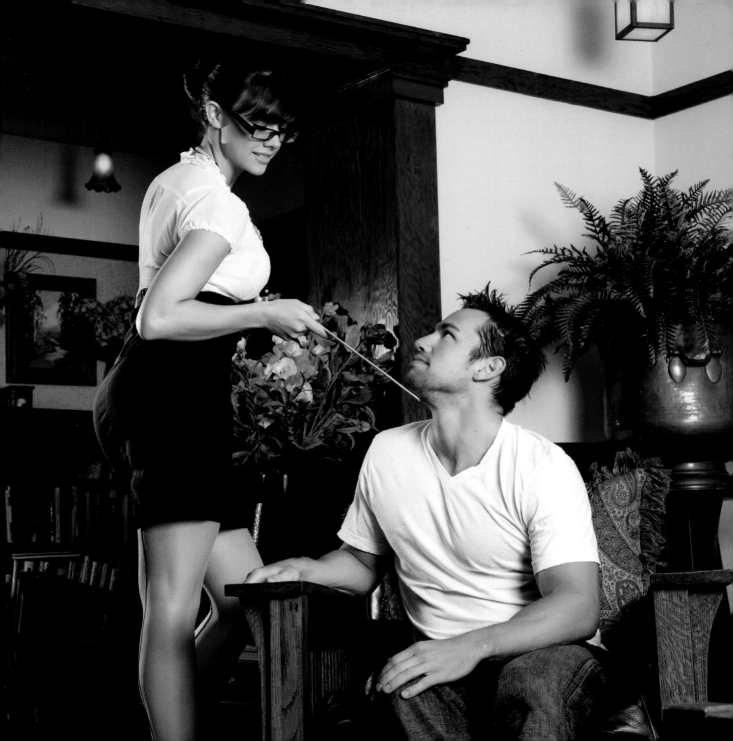

Vulva-voom!

So boys, let's set the record straight here. When people refer to girly parts, many times they refer to them as The Vagina. But the truth is that all that lovely stuff that you can see just by spreading her scrumptious thighs apart is actually the **VULVA**. The vulva includes the inner and outer lips, the perineum, the visible parts of the clitoris (see more info on that amazing organ later in this chapter), and the hairy (or waxed or shaven) mound or **MONS VENERIS** (which translates to mound of Venus, named after the goddess of love).

If you've been with a number of women, you've probably already noticed that not all vulvas look the same. In fact, there are about as many varieties of vulvas as there are varieties of women. If your experience with this unique geography is limited to porn movies and magazines, don't be fooled: Many women who display their dainty parts in public venues will do whatever it takes to give their vulva a nice, clean, uniform look. Some of them opt for vaginoplasty or labiaplasty surgeries intended to "create a more aesthetically pleasing appearance."[2] And those perfectly shaded and shaped pussies you see in *Playboy* have likely been airbrushed to appear perfectly symmetrical.

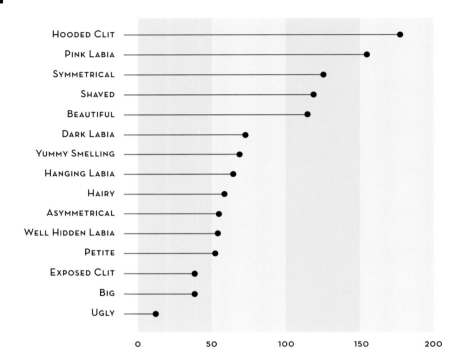

CHOOSE THE BEST TERM TO DESCRIBE YOUR VULVA

All vulvas are different. Here is how some of our survey respondents described theirs.

We reject the notion that all vulvas should look the same, and we hope that you are mature enough to love and appreciate all the shapes and sizes that exist. After all, how dull it would be if all women were identical from hair color to breast size? Encourage your woman to love what she's got and give her plenty of compliments. Says fifty-something B.K., "I always tell her how hot she is, how good she tastes, how puffy her lips are, and how sexy her engorged her clit is."

Aside from those plump and scrumptious outer lips, the waxed or gloriously bushy mound, and that cute and pleasure-sensitive little stretch of highway between her delectables and her anus (i.e., the perineum), the rest of those visible parts of the vulva actually make up the wonderland that is her clitoris. Read on.

The Vagina: VajiWOW!

So what is the vagina? Simply put, it's the holiest of all holes, and likely the source of your ultimate penis satisfaction. (Yes, boys, this is where you get to put your dick—if you're lucky!) The word *vagina* is derived from the Latin word for sheath. It's a long and flexible muscular structure that extends from the opening of the vulva (the vestibule) to the **CERVIX** (a door to the uterus that remains mostly shut except for when giving birth). Besides its role as a warm, wet place for your penis (or her favorite sex toy), it also serves as birth canal and path for menstruation. Note that much of her clitoral organ resides in the first 3 inches (7.6 centimeters) of her vaginal opening, and the nerve endings and blood vessels there are plentiful. Beyond the first third of her vagina, she has virtually zero nerve endings, which means that the area responds well to pressure, but not much else. During sex play with your girl, you would be wise to learn that it's not about how deep you can get it (although some women enjoy a little cervix bumping now and again); rather, it's about how much (and how well) you stimulate all those enervated areas in the first third of her vaginal canal and along her clitoris.

Public Primping

In 1970s porn films, the bush was big. But in 1980, porn star Marilyn Chambers trimmed her pubic hair into the shape of a heart and shaved her lips bare for her appearance in the naughty flick *Insatiable*. Thanks to the influence of the porn industry, today it's common practice for American women to tame their pubes in all manner of ways.

In our survey, 78 percent of our female respondents say they regularly shave, wax, or trim their pubic hair, and only 4 percent say that they leave it completely and naturally wild.

The latest trend is vajazzling, which is the application of glitter and jewels where pubic hair used to be. Actress Jennifer Love Hewitt admitted in her book *The Day I Shot Cupid* (2010) that she vajazzles her mound with Swarovski crystals, and in a January 2010 interview on *Lopez Tonight*, she said that her "precious lady shines like a disco ball."

BE THE CLIT COMMANDER

Think that the clitoris is just a teeny tiny little nub that pokes out from the upper part of her vulva? Think again. Traditional viewpoints hold that the clitoris has only four parts (the glans, the shaft, the crura, and the vestibular bulbs). However, the Federation of Feminist Women's Health Centers (FFWHCs), founded by Carol Downer, undertook extensive hands-on vulva research in the 1970s and determined that there are at least eighteen parts to the clitoris.[3] Modern-day sex educators echo this finding. In a 2004 interview with Paul Ford of *The Morning News*, Dr. Ian Kerner says about the clit, "It's the pleasure dome. You set one nerve moving and they all start moving. The clitoris has 18 separate parts that contribute to the experience of pleasure, twice as many nerve fibers as the penis (over 8,000), the uncanny ability to produce multiple orgasms and no known purpose other than pleasure."[4]

Gentlemen, it's time to stop thinking of the clitoris as just a small but sensitive part of her pussy and start thinking of it as a fully developed organ that is as large (it can measure up to 8 inches [about 20 centimeters] in length from commissure to fourchette) and perhaps more complex than your penis.

The Parts that Make Her Go Mmm

So what are these eighteen parts of the clitoris and what should you know about them? Here's an overview of all the pieces that add up to pleasure with a capital P.

1. The **COMMISSURE** is located at the top of her vulva, where the smooth flesh meets the fuzzy flesh of her outer lips. Applying light pressure to this area can be a great place to start indirectly stimulating the clitoral glans. When masturbating, some women will place a finger in this spot and press down or massage it in small circles. Try touching her here during your voyage and see how she responds.

2. From the commissure, travel down about ½ an inch to 1 inch (1.3 to 2.5 centimeters) to the **CLITORAL HOOD**. This small flap of skin covers the clitoral glans and is analogous to your foreskin (that is, if you're uncircumcised). A soft upward stroke with a fingertip or flick of the tongue is a nice way to introduce yourself to this morsel of flesh.

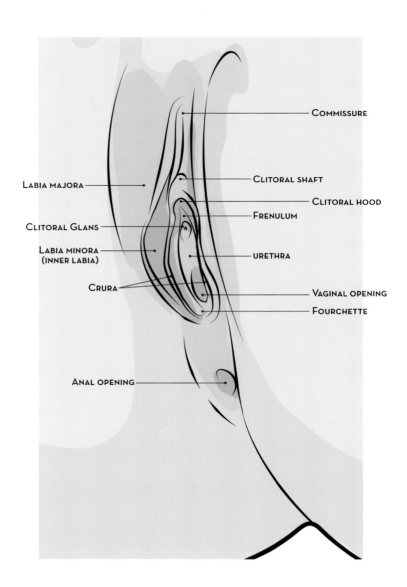

Labels:
- COMMISSURE
- CLITORAL SHAFT
- CLITORAL HOOD
- FRENULUM
- LABIA MAJORA
- CLITORAL GLANS
- URETHRA
- LABIA MINORA (INNER LABIA)
- CRURA
- VAGINAL OPENING
- FOURCHETTE
- ANAL OPENING

3. Just beneath the hood you'll find the **CLITORAL GLANS**, or the one part of the clitoris that you are likely already familiar with. The glans is somewhat analogous to the head of your penis (in fact, the two develop from the same cells in the womb). When she is excited, the glans will expand to about twice its original size and protrude from beneath the hood. When she is very near orgasm, the glans will retract once more beneath the hood.

The focal point of her clitoral orgasm, the glans is highly sensitive. Some women like direct stimulation of the nub, while others prefer you to approach this spot a little more delicately, and often indirectly, especially if your approach involves your fingertips (rather than your tongue or the thrilling meeting of your pubis to her clitoris).

4. The **FRENULUM** is a bit of connective tissue that joins the clitoral glans to the edge of the inner labia. You have a frenulum, too—it's that sensitive strip of tissue that joins your penis head to your shaft on the underside of your cock. Like yours, hers is very sensitive and may respond well to a warm, wet lick.

5. Just beneath the surface of the glans and extending back up toward the commissure, you will feel a $1/2$ to 1-inch (1.3- to 2.5-centimeter) column of flesh called the **CLITORAL SHAFT**. This is actually a piece of erectile tissue that expands when she's excited. Try rolling or gently pinching the shaft while your lady is in the throes of excitement—this is a nice way to indirectly stimulate the nerve-packed glans. Some women find that one side of the shaft is more sensitive to touch than the other—all the more reason to give your girl a close-up examination to determine whether she's a righty or a lefty.

6. The clitoral shaft forks into two legs called the **CRURA**, which travel back down the vulva just beneath her inner labia. This wishbone-shaped area is also made of erectile tissue. In effect, the crura hug the entrance to the vagina and may explain why women often report enjoying the feeling of being "stretched open" by a particularly fat cock, your splayed fingers, or a fun toy. The stretch ensures contact with the legs of her clitoris. Don't overlook this area during your oral ministrations: Several nice, long licks along the crura can be a delightful feeling, indeed.

7. The **INNER LABIA (LABIA MINORA)** are morsels of girly flesh that are highly sensitive to pleasure. When she is excited, the inner labia will swell, and as she approaches orgasm, the color will noticeably darken. These friends can clue you in to how excited your partner really is. A long, loving lick, a gentle tug, a tender massage, or tenderly pinching and rubbing them together—these are all ways to excite and arouse her labia.

8. The **G-SPOT** is a bit of female anatomy named after Dr. Ernst Gräfenberg, a gyne-cologist who first related the area to sexual pleasure.[5] The G-spot is located about 1–3 inches (2.5–7.6 centimeters) inside the vagina, along the upper side, toward the front of her body, and its texture differs from the surrounding tissue. It is the back of her clitoris and the focal point of her **URETHRAL SPONGE**. (The urethral sponge is made of spongy erectile tissue that wraps around the **URETHRA**, or the tiny hole just below the clitoral head where her urine passes through). The G-spot varies in size from woman to woman—some have a spot the size of a fingertip while others have a G-area closer to the size of a half-dollar coin. No matter the size, as the back of the nerve-rich clitoris, this area has a high density of nerve endings, and attention to this spot can lead to orgasm for some women. Other women aren't as sensitive—you'll have to experiment with yours to find out how much stimulation she likes. You can manipulate the G-spot effectively with your fingers, a sex toy, or your penis. You will feel the area become ridged, or erect, as she approaches her orgasm. (For more information on the G-spot, read Chapter 2.)

9. Embedded in the tissue of the urethral sponge and G-spot are the **PARA-URETHRAL GLANDS**, which are linked to production of alkaline fluids. The largest of these are the Skene's glands, located near the urethral opening and believed to be the source of the fluid produced during female ejaculation.[6] (For more on female ejaculation, see Chapter 2.)

10. The **FOURCHETTE** is the fork at the lower-most point of her clitoral tissue, where it meets the perineum. This spot can be a powerhouse of sexual response. Try inserting your finger (to the first knuckle) into her vaginal opening, with the pad of your finger facing down. Gently press down toward her anus, then stroke from side to side. A firm press of your tongue can also illicit a sexy response.

11. The **PERINEAL SPONGE** is located inside the bottom portion of her vaginal opening, just past the fourchette and behind the perineum. Like the urethral sponge, this is a spongy cluster of erectile tissue that becomes ridged during heightened sexual response and is responsive to your touch.

The Other Parts of Her Cutie-Pie Clit

12. The **CLITORAL BULBS** are made of two corpus cavernosa, a type of erectile tissue that fills with blood during sexual response. (You have these in your penis, too: They are the parts that fill with blood to create your erection.) The twin bulbs are located on either side of the vaginal opening, along the clitoral legs.

13. The **HYMEN** is an ultra-fragile membrane that covers all or part of the vaginal opening, but usually perforates or disintegrates by the time a woman is in her mid-teens (via a variety of causes, not just sex). Sometimes you can see the remnants of the hymen as a triangular bit of flesh just beyond the vaginal opening.

14. The **BARTHOLIN'S GLANDS** are two pea-size glands, located on either side of her inner labia, just below the vaginal opening. They produce a small amount of lubrication around the outer portion of her vulva during the later stages of her arousal.

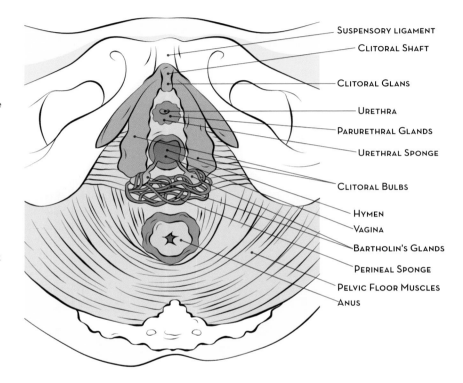

SUSPENSORY LIGAMENT
CLITORAL SHAFT
CLITORAL GLANS
URETHRA
PARURETHRAL GLANDS
URETHRAL SPONGE
CLITORAL BULBS
HYMEN
VAGINA
BARTHOLIN'S GLANDS
PERINEAL SPONGE
PELVIC FLOOR MUSCLES
ANUS

15. The **PELVIC FLOOR MUSCLES** include the **BULBOCAVERNOSUS MUSCLE**. This clitoral muscle encircles both the vagina and the anus in a figure eight shape, which is one reason why anal sex feels good to some women.[7] Other muscles that keep everything in working order include the **ISCHIOCAVERNOSUS MUSCLES**, the **TRANSVERSE PERINEAL MUSCLE**, the **ANAL SPHINCTER MUSCLES**, the **UROGENITAL DIAPHRAGM**, and the **PUBOCOCCYGEUS (PC) MUSCLE**. All of these muscles play integral parts in her sex function.

16. The **SUSPENSORY LIGAMENT** tightens during sex and is responsible for pulling the clitoral glans back beneath its hood upon orgasm. The **ROUND LIGAMENT** attaches the tissue beneath the labia minora to the uterus.

17. The **PUDENDAL NERVE** carries the pleasure sensation from the clitoris through the spinal cord to the brain. This nerve is also responsible for carrying signals from the anus and the urethra via two other branches.

18. BLOOD VESSELS are interwoven through the clitoral organ and increase blood supply. When these blood vessels are full, the walls of the vagina will sweat that slippery honey that you love so much. The arteries allow blood in, causing her erectile tissues to swell in excitement, and the veins allow blood out. However, unlike your penis, the blood flows in and out of the area more easily. This is one reason why women are able to have multiple orgasms, instead of the one ejaculatory shot you guys get before the whole system must reset.[8]

We hope that you'll put this road map to female anatomy to good use. Don't worry if you get a little lost along the way: It's okay to (*gasp!*) ask your partner for directions. Or if you're too shy (or too proud) to do that, you can always come back to this chapter to review the female road map as you make your journey toward becoming an excellent lover and a true clit-ologist.

CHAPTER 2

THE BIG O

JOURNEY TO THE CENTER OF HER ORGASM

O Toe-curling, grasping, moaning, shaking, panting, hard nipples, pelvic contractions, and a well-timed "Oh my fucking god, I'm coming!" followed by a full-bodied explosion... We all strive for this unbelievable combination of sensations in bed: the female orgasm.

While it's not your sole responsibility to deliver your partner earth-shattering orgasms, if you have any ambition whatsoever to become an amazing lover, the number one rule you should follow is: *Put her pleasure first*. Whether this results in her orgasm may depend on the day, the mood, or the woman—but by putting her pleasure first you'll be stacking the odds in favor of her experiencing a knockout, drag-out climax that will put a smile on her face (and on yours). Says Alex, a forty-something lawyer, "Her orgasm is the most exciting part of sex for me, actually. More fun than mine."

"AN ORGASM A DAY KEEPS THE DOCTOR AWAY."

– MAE WEST

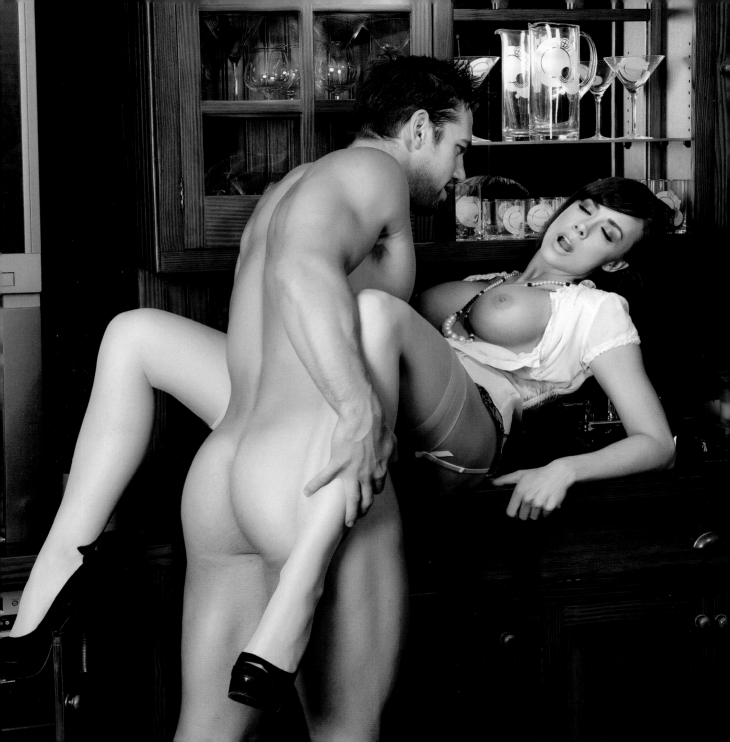

She's Wet, But Is She Ready?

Men, it's important to note that a woman's genitals are often lubricated, even when she's not aroused. Cathy Winks and Anne Semans, authors of *The Good Vibrations Guide to Sex*, write that "vaginal lubrication doesn't automatically follow sexual arousal and doesn't automatically indicate sexual arousal. Lubricating is influenced by hormonal fluctuations and can vary dramatically, depending on where a woman is in her menstrual cycle."[10] The more estrogen she produces, the wetter she'll get. And although her vagina may get nice and slippery moments after you start giving it affection, be aware that it doesn't necessarily mean that she's mentally ready to get her freak on.

Travel Time on the Road to Her Orgasm

Here's the next important thing to keep in mind: If you want to see her O face, you need to take your time. The female sexual response cycle is typically longer than yours and the building of excitement is critical to her climax. A 1994 *Sex in America* study by National Opinion Research Center at the University of Chicago found that only one out of three women typically achieved orgasm, but when they received just twenty-one minutes total of foreplay, nine of ten women were able to attain climax.[9]

In our survey, many women commented that the time it takes them to orgasm depends considerably on foreplay, which not only includes physical excitement, but a build-up of mental anticipation for a sexy event. Says forty-something S.B., "The best foreplay is verbal, and it starts from the moment you say hello."

The time it takes can also vary depending on outside factors, such as stress and environment. Says thirty-three-year-old Lily, "It depends on if I have a lot on my mind. Sometimes, I'm somewhere else and it can take longer. Or sometimes I'm just so horny and worked up it just takes a few minutes."

Gentlemen, Rev Her Engine! Vrooooooom!

In 1966, researchers William H. Masters, M.D., and Virginia E. Johnson published their groundbreaking study of human sexuality: *Human Sexual Response*. This book was a culmination of over a decade of studying men's and women's sexual patterns first hand. Masters and Johnson observed women in a laboratory setting and broke their sexual responses down into four easy phases that are still in common use in sexuality sciences today. Note that this breakdown is physiological only and does not include dinner reservations or the 10 p.m. showing of that chick flick she's been dying to see.

1. EXCITEMENT: This is the phase where she gets wet and her nipples harden. What are some things that can make her excited? Well, depending on your woman, this could include things like dirty talk; a massage; spanking; kissing; thigh, neck, and ear nibbling — you get the picture. Boys, don't make the mistake of assuming that her wetness means she's hot and ready for your cock. This is only the beginning for her, and it's best to keep her at this level of excitement for a while before diving in. You can elevate her toward the next arousal phase via oral sex, fingering, and a little toy play. To really tease and tantalize, we recommend you make it a policy to wait at least twenty minutes to initiate penetration.

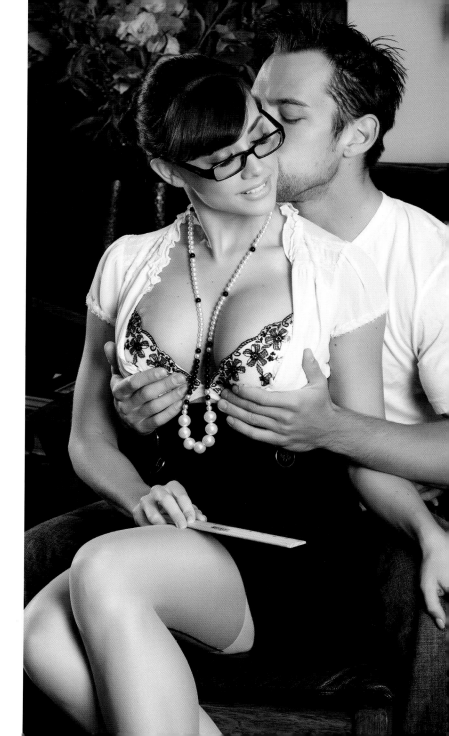

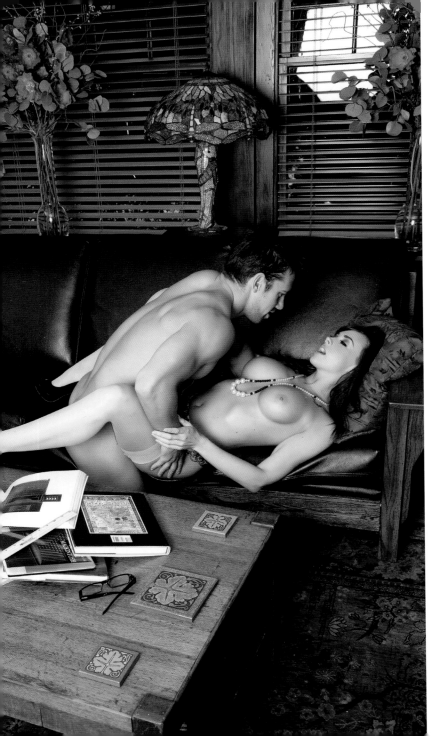

2. PLATEAU: Her labia will be puffy and red, her nipples will be painfully erect, her clitoris will withdraw into its hood, and she may actually lose some of her initial wetness. Her breathing will become rapid and her muscles will tighten. When she's in this phase, she is on the brink of orgasm, and it may just take an extra push to send her over. This is a good time to increase the intensity in your play. Depending on your woman, you could strengthen your spankings, grab her breasts, pinch her nipples, bite her neck, perform a few Kegels (tightening and releasing your pelvic muscles, which will make your cock expand inside her body) from within, thrust a little deeper and faster, introduce a vibrator, or put a finger (or toy) in her bum. You get the picture.

3. ORGASM: This is the climax of her sexual experience. This phase is evidenced by hyperventilation, muscle spasms, facial contortions, and more. (Read on for the top ten signs she's coming.) Her brain releases a delicious dose of the hormone oxytocin, which is said to bring feelings of attachment and well-being. During this phase, just hang on to your hat and don't change anything so you don't break the spell! (Be aware that some women have difficulty making the leap from plateau to orgasm, and depending on the circumstances, she may not make the leap every sexual encounter.)

4. RESOLUTION: Immediately following orgasm, her muscles and nipples will soften, and she'll collapse, completely spent. If you've got it in you, and she's willing, you can build her right back up to plateau phase and send her on another spin and possibly into a second orgasm. Or you can take the opportunity to enjoy your own climax. If she's into it, make sure you cuddle for a bit before hitting the showers. You want to make the most of her afterglow to round out the experience.[11]

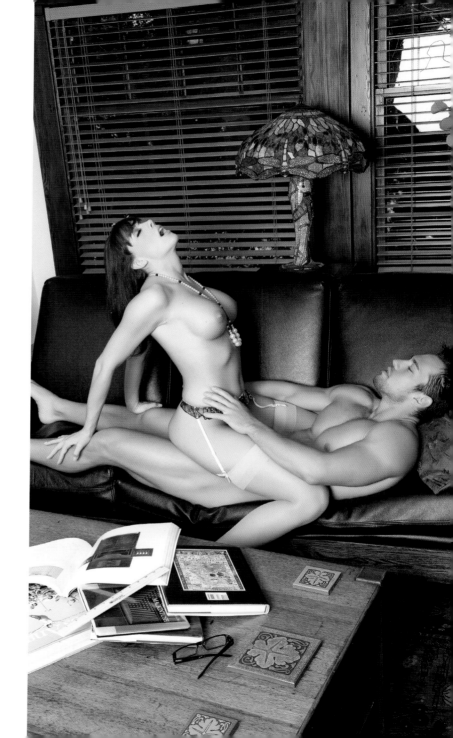

How Can You Tell If Your Partner Is Having an Orgasm?

Fifty-four percent of the men we surveyed say they can always tell when their partner is having an orgasm. (Bravo, boys! Either you are in tune with your partner's sexual response cycle, or she's mighty good at pulling the wool over your eyes.) Forty-three percent say that they can sometimes tell, and 3 percent say they have no idea when she is coming. The confusion can be caused by the variation between each woman, so it's important for you to make efforts to learn the signs that your partner exhibits. Benjamin, a twenty-four-year-old novelist says it well: "Women are like banks. Everyone has a different safe and they're not always in the same place. The digits in the combinations change from bank to bank, and, well, it's very nice when you're given the numbers instead of told to figure it out simply by touch."

Ten Signs She May Exhibit as She Experiences Climax

1. FLUSHED FACE AND CHEST: This is called a sex flush, and it makes some women red and blotchy as they approach orgasm. (Note: This is probably easier to see on an Irish lover than on a Latina lover.)

2. PULSATING AND CONTRACTIONS within her anus and pussy: This should feel extra good around your cock, tongue, or fingers.

3. EXTREME TENSION IN THE BODY: Watch for her back arching, thighs tightening, hands grasping, and facial muscles contorting. This will all be followed by abrupt relaxation and collapse after her orgasm is finished.[12]

4. (BEWARE: THESE LOUD VOCALIZATIONS DO NOT NECESSARILY MEAN ORGASM!) This is a good way to fake it (just think of the famous fake orgasm scene in the 1989 movie *When Harry Met Sally*). Not to say that women don't get loud when they come, but this is not a sure sign. Women can orgasm quietly, too. (We have practice sneaking in a masturbation session and quietly coming, too.) If she is vocal, an authentic orgasm will more likely be composed of guttural moans, crazy laughter, crying, and other illogical noises, and will not necessarily echo the self-conscious dramatics of your favorite porn star.

5. CLITORIS RETRACTION INTO THE CLITORAL HOOD AND DARK-ENING OF THE LABIA: This will be easier to see if your face is in her pussy when she comes (just another reason to practice oral sex). Technically, these signs occur during the plateau phase, about ninety seconds before the big O,[13] so now is *not* the time to change what you are doing—just keep on keepin' on.

6. INCREASE IN SIZE OF THE INNER LABIA: It may also get (even more) puffy.

7. HEART RATE PEAKS, causing her to gasp and pant, and she may break into a sweat.

8. FLOODING OR SQUIRTING if you are hitting their G-spot just right.

9. CHANGE IN TEXTURE: The flesh on the roof of her vaginal canal will sometimes become ridged or rough (something you will feel with your finger more than with your penis).

10. SHE TELLS YOU: If you're really unsure, ask her to tell you when she's coming (and to be honest) so you can really be clear about what happens when she does. Eventually you'll be familiar with her body's specific combination of reactions and you won't need the alert.

CHEAT SHEET FOR MULTIPLE ORGASMS

Eighty-three percent of our survey respondents say they've experienced multiple orgasms. Why do women get the luxury of experiencing multiple orgasms while you're stuck with only one shot? Sex therapist Dr. Jenni Skyler explains that most men typically ejaculate and orgasm at the same time, and it's the ejaculation that then necessitates a refractory, or rest, period during which his whole system needs to reset (e.g., the testicles need to make another batch of sperm). A woman's body, however, doesn't have to go through this period of rest after she orgasms because she's not ejaculating a delivery of baby batter into another person, thus her body is capable of quickly launching into another orgasm.

THE CLIT VERSES THE VAG:
WHICH O SHAKES HER TO THE CORE?

Dr. Sigmund Freud argued that vaginal orgasms were mature orgasms and therefore superior to their clitoral counterparts, thus beginning the trend of minimizing the clitoris. (Thanks a lot!) This school of thought persisted for many years and has since given many men the impression that the clitoris is a less relevant, pea-size nub, and the vagina is really where the fun is. This belief shortchanges a woman and her pleasure in myriad ways.

In the 1970s, Anne Koedt, a renowned feminist and author of *The Myth of the Vaginal Orgasm*, argued, "Although there are many areas for sexual arousal, there is only one area for sexual climax; that area is the clitoris."[14] And Dr. Albert Ellis argued that the clitoral orgasm is truth, while the vaginal orgasm is a fairy tale.[15]

Yet other researchers believe there is no difference between a clitoral and vaginal orgasm. Masters and Johnson argued that vaginal orgasms are a result of stimulation of the labia minora due to the friction of the in-and-out motion of the penis[16] (or sex toy or fingers). If we subscribe to the notion that the inner labia are part of the clitoral organ, this is in fact a clitoral orgasm, just arrived at from a different angle. Masters and Johnson wrote, "clitoral and vaginal orgasms are not separate biologic entities."[17]

THE ORGASMIC RAINBOW

Whether you choose to divide her orgasm potential in two or not, we can tell you with certainty that women experience orgasms of multiple varieties and intensities. Some they attribute to the clit and some to the vagina. The colors of the orgasmic rainbow become even more varied if you consider anal orgasms and nipplegasms (about 1 percent of women can experience orgasm via nipple stimulation alone). Moreover, some women orgasm in their sleep without any physical stimulation whatsoever[18]—a strong indicator that her orgasm is primarily linked to her brain. Here's the lesson, boys: Pay attention to more than just her vaginal canal. Her clitoris is an essential orgasm-inducing organ, as are so many other parts of her body, including her brain!

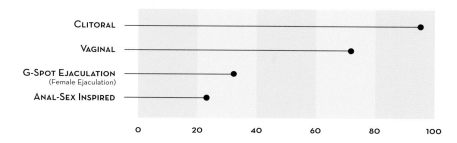

WOMEN REPORT ON WHICH TYPES OF ORGASMS THEY'VE EXPERIENCED

CLITORAL

VAGINAL

G-SPOT EJACULATION
(Female Ejaculation)

ANAL-SEX INSPIRED

0   20   40   60   80   100

Ninety-seven percent of women said they've experienced clitoral orgasms, supporting the idea that they are much easier to achieve than other types.

In our survey, 84 percent of women reported that they feel a difference between clitoral and vaginal orgasms. Says Jules, a thirty-something consultant, "A clitoral orgasm is more of a flutter, and after having one, I can come again in a very short space of time. A vaginal orgasm is much more powerful and rocks through my whole body." And Ann, a twenty-seven-year-old farmer says, "I can get off in six seconds with a clitoral orgasm. It's like eating potato chips: I'm still hungry afterward. A vaginal orgasm takes longer and is far more fulfilling. Everything shakes and trembles. I lose my damn mind." Michele, a thirty-something communications consultant, says, "Clitoral orgasm feels electrical; vaginal orgasm feels muscular. Having experienced many of both, I definitely prefer vaginal orgasms."

On the flip side, many women are champions of the clitoral orgasm. Says Meg, a twenty-five-year-old educationist, "I have never experienced a vaginal orgasm on its own, or if I have, it doesn't compare to my clitoral orgasms, which knock my socks off and last around ten to fifteen seconds!"

And Amy, a nineteen-year-old student, says, "Clitoral orgasms give me a bigger high and feel more intense. The only advantage of vaginal orgasms is that I feel closer to my partner physically and emotionally because I can feel my vaginal muscles contracting around his penis."

This is one of those debates that may never be resolved. Each woman knows her own body best, and in the end, we're all in consensus that orgasms feel amazing, no matter what!

Men Disclose on FE

Of the men we surveyed, 33 percent have been with women who have ejaculated. Here's what they had to say about the experience.

"My god, what a feeling. Incredibly warm, wet, and sloppy."
—*Jake, 34*

"I always feel honored when I can help a woman squirt. To me, it indicates a deep level of trust and comfort on her part."
—*Aaron, 42*

"It feeds my ego something awful. I imagine I feel the way women do when they receive flowers at the office."
—*Keith, 27*

"You should see our mattress. We have to use plastic sheets. I am blessed; it is not me."
—*Clarence, 54*

Thar She Blows: Female Ejaculation

Within the past decade, there has been a great deal of excitement around the G-spot and female ejaculation (FE). But as with all topics related to women's sexuality, a lot of back and forth has taken place in the scientific community about what's real and what's fantasy. The truth is, there has yet to be a definitive, scientifically sound study of FE, so we have to rely on anecdotal evidence. Going to the squirting source—that is, talking to women—makes it pretty clear that FE does indeed exist, because there are real women experiencing it.

In our survey, 33 percent of women reported having experienced FE. Says thirty-seven-year-old Sandra, stay-at-home mom, "I only had one partner who was able to do this for me. I think it was just his particular angle and size. It happened every single time. I once shot cum right into his eye. It was fantastic." Denise, a forty-two-year-old banker describes it as an "intense feeling that I am about to orgasm powerfully, followed by realizing, postorgasm, that I am absolutely soaked—I never actually feel anything spurting." Other women have a hard time putting words to the experience. Thirty-something Lily says, "They are amazing, but very difficult to experience. I don't even know how to explain—they are *that* good!"

The term *female ejaculation* is a bit misleading because different women "ejaculate" in different ways: It may result in a few teaspoons of liquid (like that little wet spot on the sheets); she may come in a flood of fluids (the gusher who needs waterproof bedding); in some cases, she may have a squirting action similar to male ejaculation; or she may produce variations of all three during different encounters, depending on her level of arousal. Some women gush at every encounter (even during quickies), while others need a lot of coaxing and gush very rarely or never.

Women experience FE in very different ways from each other (if at all!). Says thirty-something Tara, "It was clear, very much like water, and smelled like almost nothing at all." Thirty-something Denine describes her ejaculate: "I squirt enough liquid to douse my partner, my sheets, and towels, to the extent of the mattress pad being soaked. We have used a Tupperware bowl to measure my liquid, and I produce more than a cup, easily, each session." Says Ashley, a twenty-something pastry chef, about her first FE experience, "I was crouching down, using a vibrator inside, when all of a sudden, I felt my muscles contract a bit and then loosen and I felt it splash against my thighs. It was a wonderful sensation."

Another piece of the FE puzzle is the distinction between an involuntary orgasmic ejaculation and the type of ejaculation that occurs after a woman learns how to consciously gush or squirt. Most sex experts agree that FE typically occurs with continuous stimulation of the G-spot, often in conjunction with clitoral stimulation. The women who experience spontaneous, orgasmic ejaculation typically report that it feels like nothing else in this world, while women who train themselves to ejaculate report that it doesn't necessarily heighten the intensity of their orgasms.[19] (To learn more about G-spot orgasms, we recommend watching Tristan Taormino's video *Expert Guide to the G-spot*.)

SEXtracurricular Activities: Find Her Favorite Technique

By now, you've hopefully learned that every woman is unique when it comes to what makes her come. Have her complete this quick questionnaire for you and keep it handy for the next time you both get hot and bothered. We recommend giving it to her in a fun and fanciful way—for example, hide it as a "prize" in her box of cereal, and when she finds it, smile at her adoringly from across the table.

1. What is your number one sexy fantasy you'd like to see come true with me?

2. What is the best way for me to help you orgasm?

3. What are the top three most sensitive spots on your body, and how would you like for me to touch them?

Cheat Sheet:
The Journey to Female Ejaculation

If you're feeling inspired and would like to use your hand (and/or other body parts) to help your lover experience FE, here are a few techniques that might just have her squirting in your eye. (Don't forget your safety goggles!)

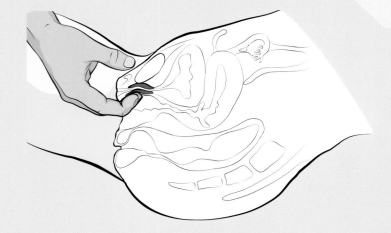

1. WARM HER UP. The tissue of the G-spot is sensitive, so it will be more receptive to pleasure when she is adequately aroused and her genitals are engorged with blood. If you try to stimulate her G-spot too soon, you could just end up irritating her! So begin with all of her favorite foreplay techniques, including kissing, nipple licking, and even some hot cunnilingus. Wait until she's thrusting and thrashing in your arms—then dip into that pot of gold.

2. LOCATION, LOCATION, LOCATION. You can't help her ejaculate if you don't know where her G-spot is! Insert your finger pad-side-up toward the front of her body. About 1–3 inches (2.5–7.6 centimeters) in you'll find a patch of tissue the texture of which is rougher than the smooth tissue surrounding it. Lightly tap it with your finger, or try rubbing the area in soft, small circles. If she likes it and wants more, rub your finger up and down more vigorously.

3. TRY A G-SPOT TOY. There are numerous toys on the market specifically meant to stimulate the G-spot. These are shaped with a slight angular bend at the top and a wide flare that is intended to massage the spot. Using a toy will save your fingers from getting fatigued, as it can take a lot of pressure and stimulation to coax a girl to erupt. Unlike the clitoral glans, the G-spot responds well to consistent and direct stimulation, and this is often best achieved with a toy.

4. PICK YOUR POSITION. If you're trying to get her to ejaculate during intercourse, it's best to warm her up with a toy and then move into a sex position where the head of your penis will rub against the front wall of her vagina. Try having her squat on top and ride a bit forward on your pelvis (see photo), or have her lie on her stomach and enter her from behind. (For more information on how to stimulate the G-spot, read Chapter 3.)

5. IT'S NOT PEE! A woman may hold back because the moment before she gushes, she feels as if she needs to pee. The fluid produced when a woman experiences the involuntary orgasmic ejaculation has been chemically analyzed and is distinct from urine in its composition.[20] This ejaculatory fluid is clear and alkaline, and originates in the Skene's glands, in the area of the spongy tissue that surrounds the urethra.[21] Says Lara,

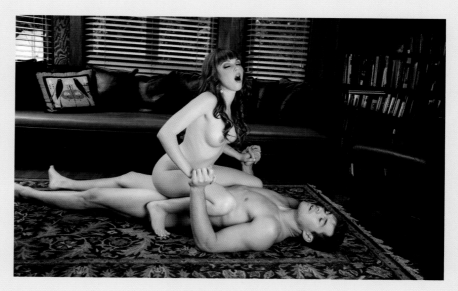

a forty-something archaeologist, "My first experience with FE was with my first lover, and he was convinced I had peed in the bed, but we both got down and sniffed the sheets and realized it wasn't pee."

Remember, many women may never experience FE, so look at your attempts to get her there as a playful and arousing journey, rather than a laborious, goal-oriented marathon. If it feels good to her, keep on touching her there, but don't worry if the G-spot stroke doesn't culminate in explosive waterworks. If it turns out that your girl is a gusher, don't forget to stock up on extra towels—or even waterproof sheets—for next time!

It's likely that each woman you meet will have her own set of instructions to bring her to climax. While one woman might advise you to talk dirty and be rough, your next partner may need you to be languorous and loving. The best thing to do is communicate with her and observe exactly what it is that gets your particular lady going. Once you've got the combination down, you'll be free to explore alternative avenues to her ultimate pleasure. Happy O hunting!

CHAPTER 3

FINGER FUN

LET YOUR FINGERS DO THE WALKING!

Men, don't make the mistake of thinking that fingering is only a prelude to intercourse. (Don't worry, you'll get your turn.) Yes, it can make for some fantastic foreplay, but the application of finger to puss can also serve as a delicious main course. Ninety-one percent of the women we surveyed tell us that they enjoy being fingered. And 19 percent say that fingering is the most reliable way for them to be brought to orgasm. That's about one out of four women—not a number to be balked at by any means. Says Bea, a twenty-something environmentalist, "It's the only way I've been able to orgasm with a partner, so I love it."

Your dexterous digits just might become some of her very best friends. If you learn how to use your fingers properly, you'll easily become the driver of her desire, her sexual response, and, if you so choose, her orgasm.

> "GIVE A MAN A FREE HAND AND HE'LL RUN IT ALL OVER YOU."
>
> – MAE WEST

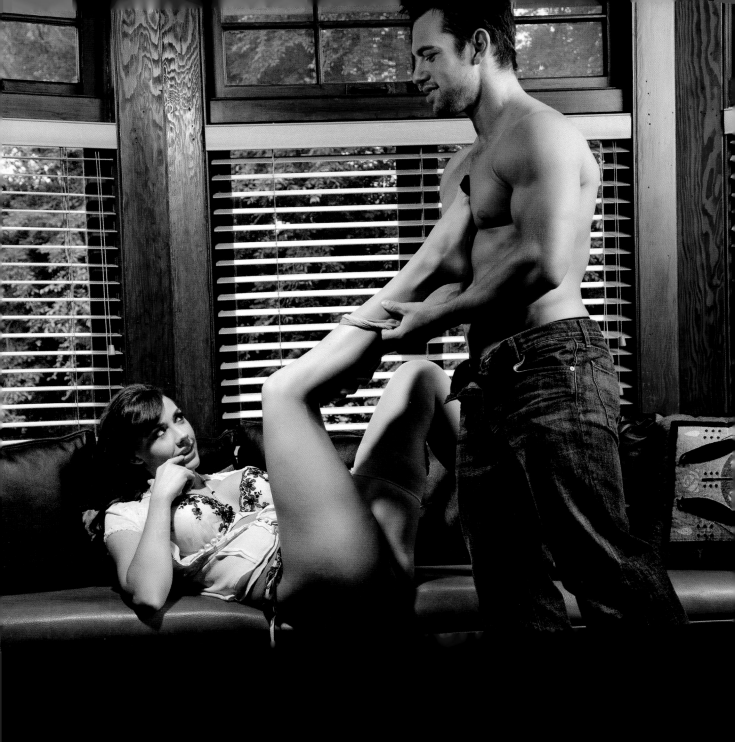

Top Six Reasons Why Fingering Can Be Better Than Fucking

Says Anne, a twenty-six-year-old writer, "I tend to enjoy being fingered better than oral sex, maybe because I enjoy G-spot orgasms more than just outer stimulation." And Hayley a twenty-year-old student says, "I like being fingered a lot better than someone going down on me. And sometimes it can even be better than actual intercourse." How could this be, you wonder? Well, here are the top six reasons why fingering rules!

1. MANEUVERABILITY: Fingers are agile and much more maneuverable than the penis. They can reach hidden spots (hello, the G-spot!), and you can intentionally deliver great pleasure to the clitoris, labia, vaginal opening, and, should she so desire, the anus—all simultaneously! Dave, a thirty-year-old engineer, says, "My fingers can give so many different sensations—they are the Swiss army knives of sex."

2. VERSATILITY: While your fingers do the walking, let your mouth play in other ways. You can kiss, nibble, lick, and bite on her neck, thighs, breasts, or even her pussy as you stroke her into a frenzy. You can also practice the art of dirty talk while you touch her (something much harder to do while your mouth is wrapped around her clit). Says Amanda, a twenty-year-old interpreter, "For me the fun in fingering is all about the dirty talk."

3. NO SELF-CONSCIOUS FACTOR: While a girl might get shy with your tongue and nose all up in her nether region, it's rare for her to feel bashful about your blind, deaf, and dumb little fingers mucking about in her stuff. "I love it, never feel self-conscious about it, and it excites me," says Nancy, a thirty-something waitress.

4. EXTENDED PLAYTIME: Unlike intercourse, the goal of fingering isn't penetration and your inevitable ejaculation. Fingering extends playtime and helps her get some extra pleasure before your greedy penis takes command of the horny ship. Says Tryna, a thirty-year-old office manager, "After my husband's vasectomy, he was instructed to not have sex for a while. During this time I experienced what I consider to be the best sex of our relationship! He fingered me to multiple orgasms, and I had the exhilarating experience of the pleasure of him not rushing toward his end goal of ejaculation."

5. CAN GO PUBLIC:

No sex act is as easy to surreptitiously take into public locations as the act of finger play. You can bury your diddling digits into her dainty drawers in a multitude of exciting and sexy locations outside of the bedroom. Says Kitty, a fifty-something massage therapist, "My partner fingers me at random times like while driving in the car, or at a restaurant, or while I'm cooking or cleaning up dishes. It's very erotic."

6. KEEPS HER GOING:

When a gentleman is working on his ejaculatory control, sometimes the moment when he has to stop thrusting so he doesn't climax too soon can be a frustrating moment for his potentially multiorgasmic partner. (Hey buddy, we're not trying to hold back *our* orgasms here!) A good way to keep her going while you're trying to lasso in your bucking bronco is to pull out of her during sex and replace your dick with one or two of your fingers and stick to the rhythm that had her going. When you've got everything back under control (i.e., you're not going to blow just yet), just get back in the saddle again.

Adding your fingers to the mix can also work wonders during those in-between moments when you're in the mood to pull an all-night sexathon. Says Lily, a thirty-something retail worker, "Fingering is awesome in my book. Sometimes we use it after he comes and we are waiting for him to get hard again for another go around."

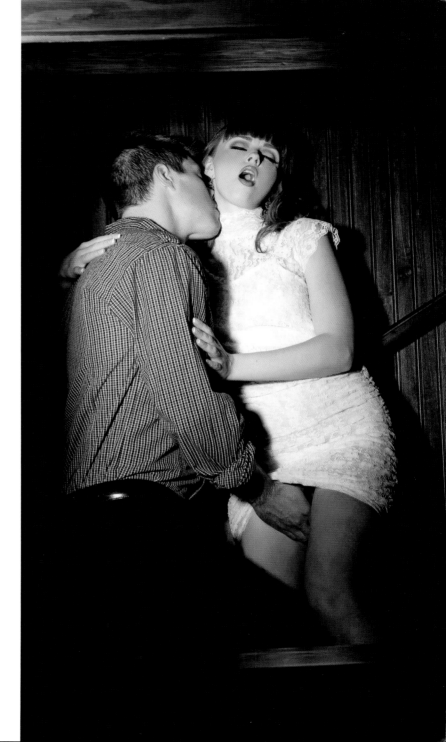

Rules of Engagement

Sure, you've probably been fingering girls ever since they first allowed you to put your hands in their shorts. But now that you are trying to get your Ph.D. in clit-ology, let's review the rules of engagement, shall we?

1. KEEP YOUR NAILS TRIMMED AND CLEANED. This the number one rule for fingering. Sharp objects do not belong on the delicate flesh of the vulva or in the vagina (unless she enjoys a little pain, but even then, she's probably thinking about something along the lines of a clit clamp, not claw marks). And because you are putting your paws inside her body, you'll want those puppies to be nice and clean.

2. BE GENTLE WITH THE CLIT—unless instructed otherwise, that is! It's easier to start out gentle and add pressure if she so desires. But if you start out rough and accidentally hurt her, she'll likely snap her legs shut and turn on the nightly news. Says Emmaline, a twenty-year-old art historian, "My clit is not a game show buzzer. Pressing it in a painful and repeated manner does not make it go off."

3. TEASE BEFORE YOU PLEASE. Don't insert your fingers into her vagina until she is wet and lubricated. (We hope you extend her this same courtesy when penetrating her with your penis.) To get her wet and ready, gently massage, kiss, and touch all of those sensitive areas on the *outside* of her pussy, including the labia, the mons, her inner thighs, and the flesh around her clit. When she is wet and aroused, add to the mix of sensations by penetrating her with your fingers. Says Vanessa, a twenty-four-year-old college grad, "Get her extremely excited and wet before entering her... There's nothing like finally feeling a finger inside my pussy after my man has been teasing me for a while."

4. REMEMBER THAT EVERY WOMAN IS DIFFERENT. This is true for every aspect of her sexual (and nonsexual) desires. A lot of the women we surveyed said they prefer a guy to start out with the clit and proceed to insertion, while other women said to save the clit for last. Says Ariana, a twenty-two-year-old flight attendant, "Don't just do it the way your ex-girlfriend liked it. Figure out what I like by experimenting."

Also note that a woman may need different speeds and pressures at different points during sex play. Some may want you to start soft and increase pressure and speed along with her building arousal, while others may prefer a more consistent touch from start to finish. What's the best way to understand your partner's preferences? Talk to her, of course. Or if you're feeling more adventurous, have her masturbate for you to show you how she likes it.

5. KNOW WHEN *NOT* TO STOP. If your goal is to send your lady to orgasmland on the tip of your fingers, this is an important rule. (Actually, this is a quintessential rule for any technique you use when she's about to come.) The closer she gets to having an orgasm, the more important it is for you to not change a single thing that you're doing, sometimes even the smallest change will send her completely off course, and you'll have to start all over again.

CHEAT SHEET: FINGER FUN

Now that we've got the rules covered, it's time for you to learn some of the sexiest, surefire techniques to wrap your woman around your finger.

1. STROKING THE STRIATIONS OF THE VULVA: Gently squeeze her outer lips together and use a very slight pinching motion to massage the flesh of her inner lips with the flesh of her outer lips. Or stroke your lady's inner labia with the pads of your fingers from top to bottom, or bottom to top. A little tug on those cute lips can also make for some sexy sensations.

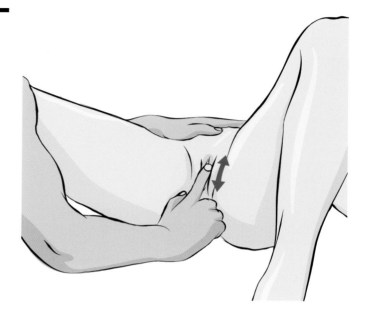

2. STRUMMING THE CLIT: From a soft tap to a circular swirl and even a light pinch, there are many ways to rock her world. As we've mentioned, the clitoral head has thousands of nerve endings and should be treated with care. A lot of women find that one side of their clitoral bulb is more sensitive than the other, or they prefer slight pressure from the top or bottom, so a fun exercise is to gently press and rub that little nub in a small circle and ask her which spot is the sweet spot. If you do it slow enough, you may not even need to ask—her gasping will tell you all you need to know.

3. FINGER FUCKING: Some women just love the simulation of a good fucking done properly with your fingers. Because of the musculature of your fingers, and the fact that you can vary the angle with which you stroke her as well as how many fingers you use, fingering can often feel more intense than intercourse.

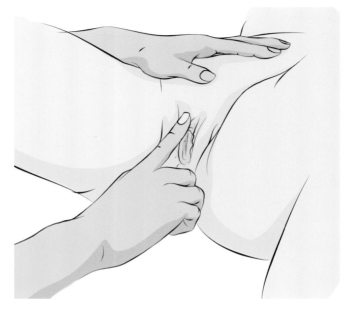

Strumming the clit

CHEAT SHEET:
FINGER FUCKING DONE RIGHT

Gentlemen, when engaging in finger fucking, always make sure your hands are clean, and don't be afraid to use a little lube. Here are a few penetrative techniques to try when you have her wet and wanting.

- Start with one finger and go slow. Think of this first penetration as exploratory. Notice how she clenches around you, and pay attention to her moans and thrusts. Twirl your finger in a circular motion to feel the outer confines of her pussy, and then slide your finger slowly in and out of her. Intersperse your finger thrusting with rubs on her clitoris.

- Insert a second finger (usually you'll use your fore and middle fingers). This will increase the pressure inside of her, and as you thrust in and out, be sure to rub up against her G-spot.

- Some women love a little G-spot knocking. Rest your palm on her mound and tap or knock your fingers up and down on her G-spot. This will be an incredibly intense sensation for her—she may clench her legs around your hand. Add to the feeling by licking her nipples. As long as you're not hurting her, keep at it—this is often a good way to make her come.

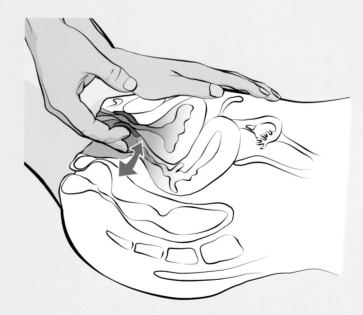

- Try stretching your fingers apart in a V shape as you slowly push them in and out of her vagina.

- If she likes the V, she may enjoy a third or even a fourth finger. The more fingers you use, the more pressure she'll feel inside. Using more fingers will fill her up in a way that your cock simply can't, because you can spread your fingers apart as you thrust into her.

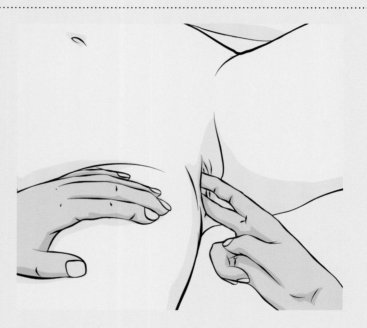

4. THE G-SPOT STROKE: Locate her G-spot and stroke her with a "come hither" motion, rubbing the area from top to bottom. For a delightful twist, rotate your fingers around the area in a tight, circular stroke. Some women will only require the lightest of touches in order to find great pleasure. Other women may need firm pressure and rapid stroking to reap the rewards. You'll know you're doing something right if she starts moaning and bucking against your hand. Also, as she approaches orgasm, you'll feel the ridges of the G-spot raise, and it will become even more textured than it was before—a dead give away that you should keep on going until she gets off.

5. TRIPLE THREAT: You don't have ten penises, but you do have ten fingers, so put them to good use and employ the triple threat. Says Kay, a fifty-year-old marketing executive, "Try hitting all three spots at once: the clit, vagina, and rectum—this may take some practice, but can be done with one hand and different fingers." Lie so that you are facing her, torso to torso (on top or on your side), insert your index and/or middle finger into her vagina, apply your thumb to her clit, and your ring finger or pinky finger can caress her anus.

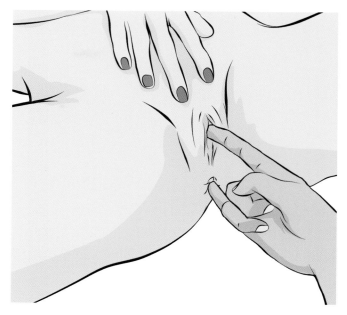

Triple Threat

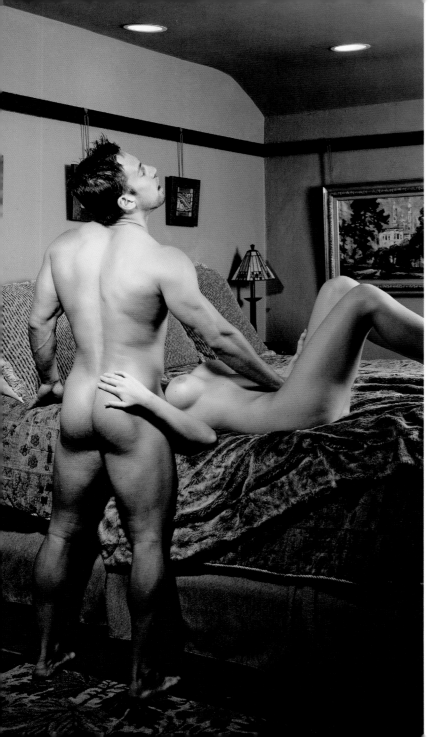

Fun Finger Positions

Yes, as with all sex acts, positions are an important consideration when giving your partner a tantalizing tickle. Says John, a forty-two-year-old math teacher, "In my opinion, a man's hands should be used more often than anything else, from a variety of angles and in a number of sexual positions."

Here are four positions that you should consider adding to your five-digit dance routine.

1. WRAP-AROUND

Want to touch her like she touches herself? To get the appropriate angle, sit behind her and wrap your arms around her torso. Use one hand to stroke her labia and the inside of her vagina, and the other to tease and tantalize her clit.

« 2. ON THE EDGE

Have your woman lie on her back along the edge of the bed. Stand alongside her and finger her with one hand and massage her breasts with the other. Added bonus: If she turns her head to the side and you position yourself right, she can lick and suck on your cock while you touch her sweet spot.

3. UP CLOSE AND PERSONAL »

Lie side by side, facing each other on the bed. Wrap your bottom arm around your lady and pull her close into a kiss. Massage her back or the nape of her neck. Reach between your bodies with the other hand and undulate your fingers between her folds. This is a good angle to use the clamp technique, wherein you put your first two fingers into her vagina, and use your thumb to rub her clitoris—your fingers and thumb will make the shape of a clamp. Just be mindful not to clamp down and apply too much pressure on the clit!

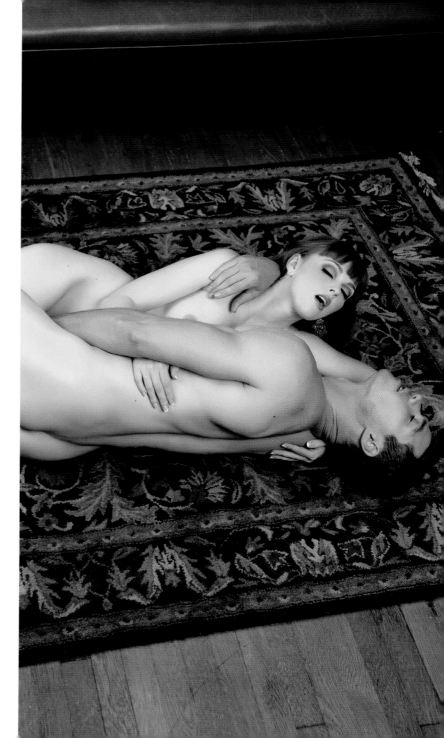

4. FROM BEHIND »

Have her get on all fours or lie on her stomach, then kiss and nibble on the back of her neck. Gently slide your thumb inside her and massage her G-spot. Use your other fingers to tantalize her clitoris or breasts.

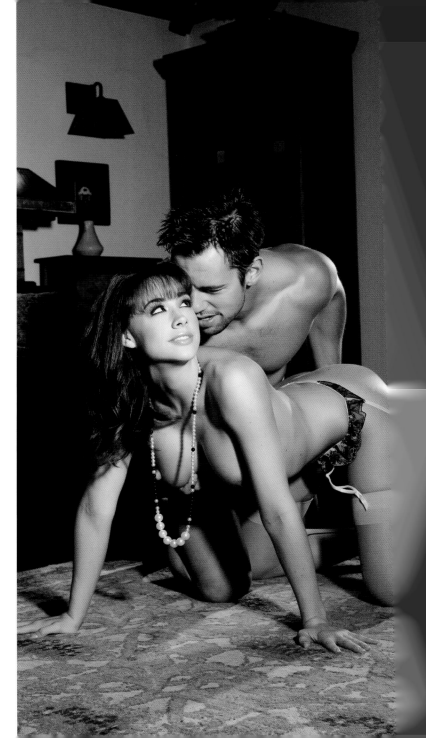

SEXtracurricular Activities: Watch and Learn

Your woman knows best when it comes to touching herself. This is your opportunity to encourage her to show you firsthand how she likes it done.

. . . .

1. THE SET-UP: While you are hot and heavy and she's already wet and super-excited, tell her in your sexiest bad-boy voice that you want her to show you how to touch her. Take her hand and guide it to her pussy and tell her to touch herself for you.

2. PAY ATTENTION: Watch what parts of herself she touches. Does she spend her time massaging her clit? Does she dip a finger or two inside? Does she rest one hand on her pubic bone while she touches, or does she put both hands to work simultaneously? Ask her to talk you through her methods.

3. ENCOURAGE HER: Like the naughty coach you are, encourage her to continue. Tell her how hot she looks, entreat her to keep going, and assure her you've never seen anything so sexy in your life. This will give her the confidence she needs to let her inner exhibitionist out.

4. SHOW HER WHAT YOU'VE LEARNED: When you simply can't keep your hands off of her anymore, gently replace her hands with yours. Try to match her actions touch for touch and truly get a feel for what your sexy lady likes. If she'd like, ask her to guide your hands or describe what's working as you work your hands on her pussy.

Fisting: Stretch Her to the Limit

Fisting (also known as fist fucking) is the act of inserting all five fingers and hand into the vagina. This move is for the über-adventurous and requires patience, practice, and enthusiasm. Only 5 percent of our respondents said they love being fisted, while 36 percent were curious to try it. Says forty-something Deedee, "Fisting is very stimulating for me, and it reliably brings me to orgasm."

When done correctly, fisting can be an amazingly pleasurable sex act—the stretching feeling pressing against the clitoral crura, the ultimate surrender and relaxation that it requires from her, and the titillating sensations of your knuckles rubbing up against that very sensitive flesh in the front third of her vagina all add up to *wow!*

Follow these rules of fisting to ensure a sexy and fun experience.

1. LUBRICATE, LUBRICATE, LUBRICATE. She needs to be as slippery as a Minnesota sidewalk in January. So apply generous portions of water-based lubricant to your hands and her vaginal opening.

2. START CLEAN. You don't want to push your dirty mitts into her vagina, so make sure your hands are clean and your fingernails are trimmed. Wearing latex gloves can help make your hand slide in smoothly and keep things sterile and safe. And no jewelry!

3. MAKE SURE SHE'S RELAXED. She needs to be fully open and receptive to the act. If she's tense and unsure, her whole body will tense up and fisting will be impossible. A nice hot bath, a massage, and a lot of fun sex play before you try to fill her up will help her get into that relaxed and receptive state.

4. STRETCH HER SLOWLY. Start with one finger, then two, and as she relaxes, three, then four fingers. All the while, work on gently stretching her vaginal opening by massaging it in circles. Once all four fingers are in, gently position your thumb beneath your fingers and maneuver it forward and inside. This leaves just the widest part of your hand to go in—and yes, it does. Thus the name fisting. As you penetrate her with your hand, keep it in a beak shape so that it is as narrow as possible and continue to apply lubrication generously. If she's excited enough, her vagina will suck your hand right in.

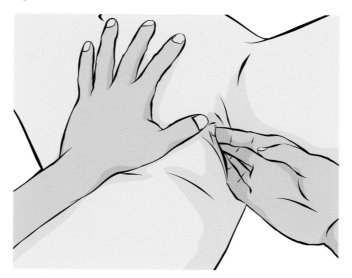

5. COMMUNICATE. Make sure you constantly communicate with your partner, both verbally and by watching her body language. Make sure she is comfortable as you insert each additional finger and finally your fist.

Often, the best sex can be had when you use everything at your disposal, including your hands, to please your partner. If you learn nothing else from this book, learn this: By pleasing your partner, you'll be able to reap the rewards of the hottest, sexiest sex you'll ever have.

CHAPTER 4

LICKING THE CUNNY

PROPER TECHNIQUES FOR DELIVERING AMAZING CUNNILINGUS

Gentlemen, when it comes to being an amazing lover to your lady, there is just nothing like knowing how to give her good oral sex. Arguments and annoyances can be easily forgiven if you are a stellar cunnilinguist. Just how many licks does it take to get to the center of her orgasm? It depends on the woman, of course! But rest assured, almost all women enjoy your mouth on her private parts (78 percent of our survey respondents said they do), and nothing sounds as sweet as a sincere "Mmm, you taste so good."

Many women report that there is nothing as intense as having an orgasm via oral sex. According to *The Hite Report: A Nationwide Study of Female Sexuality* (2004), 42 percent of women orgasm regularly during cunnilingus.[22] Our survey numbers are similar: 36 percent of our female respondents report that they always orgasm during oral sex, and another 47 percent say that they sometimes do.

Dr. Jenni says, "Cunnilingus can offer women the ability to completely relax. She's in the pleasure seat, and she can just receive. Ultimately, she can completely surrender. And orgasm is all about surrender."

"WHEN IT COMES TO PLEASURING WOMEN AND CONVERSING IN THE LANGUAGE OF LOVE, CUNNILINGUS SHOULD BE EVERY MAN'S NATIVE TONGUE."

– IAN KERNER,
SHE COMES FIRST

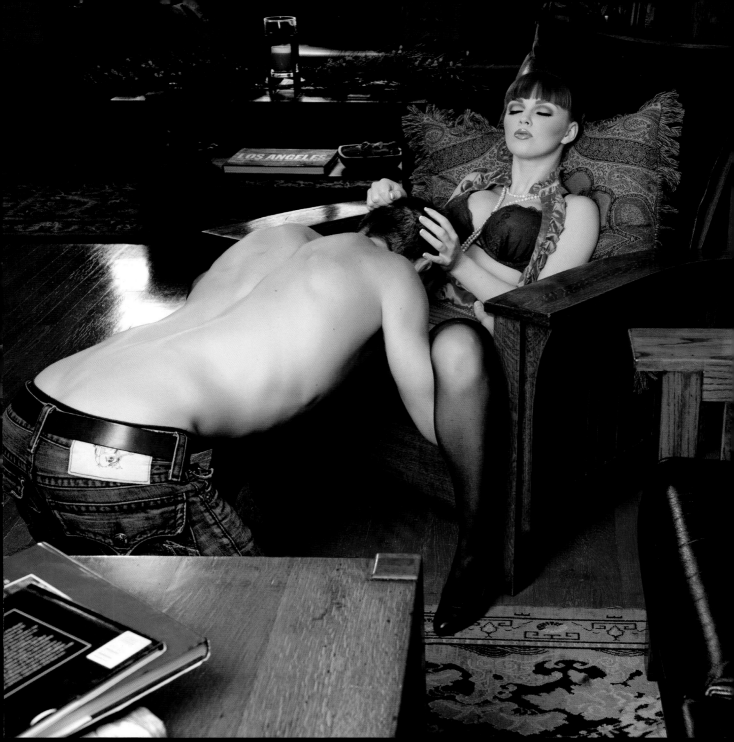

THE VULVA IS A WONDERFUL THING TO TASTE

You can learn all the pussy-pleasing techniques in this book, but it won't get you anywhere without proper understanding of the relationship between her pleasure and her mind-set. To get to the point where you can unzip her and lick her, you'll need to approach her with the right attitude and overcome any inhibitions she may have.

Women can be extremely self-conscious about receiving cunnilingus. They worry that they might smell bad or look strange or unappealing down there, or they may be too embarrassed to orgasm in your face. Says Amanda, a twenty-something interpreter, "I'm quite self-conscious about the whole thing. I enjoy the feeling of it, but have not yet been able to let go enough to orgasm that way." Twenty-four-year-old Darian says, "It feels good, but there is often a degree of self-consciousness. I'm always afraid I will smell or be unpleasant for my partner, even though I've always been told it smells good."

So gentlemen, how do you handle your tongue-shy minx? Here are some tips for helping your lovely lady to open up and, hopefully, blossom into orgasm under your oral techniques.

COMPLIMENTS ARE KEY

Just as she loves it when you tell her how amazing she looks in that dress, talking up her pussy will earn you points. Some good key phrases to learn include: "You taste so good; I could eat you up all day" and "God, your pussy is beautiful." Says 44-year-old Chuck, "I love the look and feel of her lips, and how she smells, and the curves of her mons, and I tell her so all the time." The important thing here is, you really need to be sincere about what you are saying. If you tell her that she tastes yummy, but then screw up your nose and only lick her a couple of times before coming up for air, chances are she'll never feel comfortable with you going down on her again.

Engage in Watery Fun to Get Her Wet!

A lot of women will be more relaxed about receiving cunnilingus if they are absolutely positive that they're squeaky clean. So why not jump in the shower or bath together? You can suds her up and use a finger or two to stroke her clitoris or gently finger fuck her. Be careful about using soaps or bath products on and especially *inside* the pussy. Her pH balance is extremely delicate and you could unwittingly give your lady a nasty irritation or infection. Warm water and a gentle washing will leave her sweet and lickably clean. Then you can lead her wet, naked body to the bed for some lickin' and lovin'. Alternatively, she may feel more comfortable freshening up on her own. No matter how she gets clean, everyone agrees cleanliness can add a huge dose of confidence to any love-making session!

Set the Mood

Make sure the environment is primed for her sexual relaxation. Turn off the TV, make the bed (if it's not already made), and light a few candles. The mellow, dimly lit room will make her feel comfortable, especially if she's shy, and the absence of twisted, crumpled sheets and that pesky sitcom dialogue in the background will make her feel like it's all about her.

Take Your Time

If you're like a lot of guys, giving oral sex can be such a turn-on that your penis wants to take over the job sooner than later. Try to resist your dick's selfish ways. While a warm, wet mouth and a few tongue strokes can bring most men to the edge, women usually take quite a bit longer than men to reach orgasm. If you do a rush job, you may give her the idea that you're not really into it and you probably won't lead her to orgasm (or even to the brink).

Don't Let Her Give Up Too Soon

Often, when a self-conscious woman is on the receiving end of oral sex, she might hesitate to actually orgasm with your face between her legs. This means that when she's close—and we mean really close—she just might try to get away. It's time to use a firm but gentle approach here and insist she keep her (lower) lips locked to yours as she approaches free fall. At this point, it is crucial that you do *not* change your stroke. Hopefully, you'll be able to coax her through her inner turmoil so that she can come out the other side with a blissful grin on her face and the belief that you are the best lover *ever*.

Cheat Sheet: Pussy Comes in Many Flavors

Of the men we surveyed, 12 percent said their partner's pussy tasted like a particular food item. Here were some of the foods they used for comparison:

- A seafood platter
- Apple
- Blueberries
- Cantaloupe
- Caramel ice cream
- Cherry pie
- Chocolate
- Echinacea (herbal tea)
- Garlic (we had just eaten Thai food)
- Honey
- Lemon
- Licorice
- Melon
- Onions
- Oysters
- Peaches
- Peppermint Lifesaver
- Pineapple
- Sherry
- Strawberries
- Sweet cream
- Tropical fruit
- Vanilla
- Water
- Wine

From Fresh Fruit to Heavenly and Heady, the Many Flavors of your Lover

The taste and smell of a woman's pussy varies from day to day (and of course, each woman tastes and smells different from the next). Her smell and flavor can be affected by a wide range of factors, from her hormonal cycle or state of sexual arousal to her vaginal health, her diet, how much water she drinks, the vitamins she takes, her stress levels, her birth control, and sometimes even the clothes she wears.

She Is What She Eats

Diet appears to be a mitigating factor in the way your lover smells and tastes. Of the women we surveyed, 32 percent said that their odor and (reported) flavor changed based on their diet. Similarly, 27 percent of men said their partner's diet seemed to affect her flavor and smell. Says Dale, a thirty-six-year-old accountant, "Berries or fruit seem to make her taste sweeter. When we have eaten heavier foods, like fats and garlic, there is a somewhat stronger flavor. I actually enjoy a stronger-flavored pussy; it gets me even more aroused, if that is possible." Henry, a twenty-four-year-old mechanic, notes, "Her taste changes especially after eating seafood (prawns) and some spices (especially garlic, fenugreek, and cardamom)."

It stands to reason that foods that affect the smell of urine and sweat can affect the smell of and taste of her sexual secretions, as well. Such foods include garlic, asparagus, coffee, curry, and onions. Says thirty-seven-year-old Layla, "I'm a huge coffee fiend, and my boyfriend says he can taste it down there—not too bad, actually!" Taking a multivitamin can also change her smell and flavor. And a woman who is well-hydrated tends to smell and taste slightly milder than when she's dehydrated.

To keep her vagina wet, sweet-smelling, and healthy, she should drink plenty of water and eat plenty of fruits, vegetables, and legumes, which prevent both yeast and bacterial infections.

Cheat Sheet: Cunnilingus

Okay, now that you've mastered the appropriate attitude and have developed a taste for pussy, it's time to get busy pleasing your lady. Here is a handy cheat sheet to help you make your best impression.

1. THE LONG LAP: Flatten your tongue into a wide plane (think of a dog panting in the heat) and simply lap upward, from the vestibule to the clitoris. This is a good move to start with, as it sets the stage by essentially saying "I want to taste all of you!" It's also a good transition move. And the wet warmth of your tongue will feel amazing on her labia.

2. THE TICKLE LICK: Many women enjoy a soft, light lick rather than a hard, ravenous one. Keeping your tongue soft and supple, use the tip to give her featherlike licks up and down on her clitoris and the surrounding area. You can start out slowly and then pick up speed as she gets more wound up. However, don't increase pressure as you increase your speed unless she asks you to.

3. THE GENTLE PRESS: With the front third of your tongue, gently press on her clitoral glans and intersperse this with small, fluttering licks. This move will give her just the right balance of pressure and tease—it's a great way to build her into a frenzy.

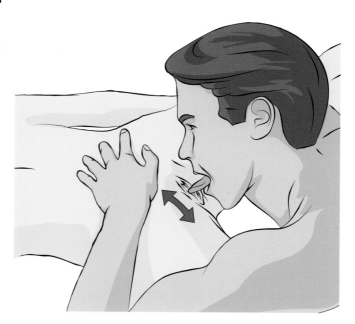

The Long Lap

4. THE HARD LICK: If your girl does prefer pressure on her clitoris, you may have to get that tongue in shape! Point it firmly and see how hard you can lick up and down and side to side on her vulva and clit.

5. THE SWIRL: Use the tip of your tongue to make a circular, swirling motion around her clit. You can expand the swirl to touch more of the vulva, and then tighten it up again on her tiny nub. Try different speeds and pressures. This is a good move for building pleasure, and you may also find that a certain size swirl will actually be your go-to move to bring her to climax.

6. THE TAP-IN: Feel free to tap in a partner for your tongue—your fingers, of course! Slowly strum her G-spot as you lick her clit. Or, if she asks for more, give her a nice, assertive finger fuck as you lap her to climax.

7. THE KINKY TAP-IN: For an extra-kinky twist, penetrate her with a dildo or vibrator as you go down. For an extra-extra-kinky twist, simply press your finger to her asshole. This may just be the special something she needs to climax. You can even insert your finger into her anus. You probably won't need to push very deep to provide the desired stimulation.

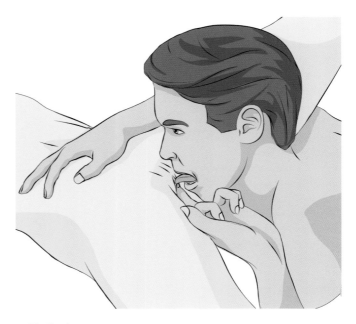

The Tap-In

8. THE SNEAK: For some women, the clitoral glans is super-duper sensitive and can't handle direct stimulation, so you might need to apply an indirect approach. Use your hot breath to caress the nub. Add gentle touches around, but not on, this ultra-sensitive spot.

9. THE NIBBLE: Use your teeth to nibble (not bite!) the flesh of her outer labia, her lower stomach, and her inner thighs. If you want to try to touch your teeth to her inner labia, be extra careful and hold the delicate flesh between your teeth as you gently pull them down and away from her vaginal opening. Follow any bites with gentle licks and kisses.

10. THE HOOVER: Form a suction cup with your lips around her clitoral glans or her inner labia and give the flesh a nice long suck just as if you were sucking your thumb. Let it audibly pop out of your mouth and follow the suck with a gentle lick before going back for more.

11. THE TONGUE FUCK: Use a stiff tongue to dart in and out of her vaginal opening. This move will make her feel like there is a smaller, wetter, more succulent dick caressing her cunt.

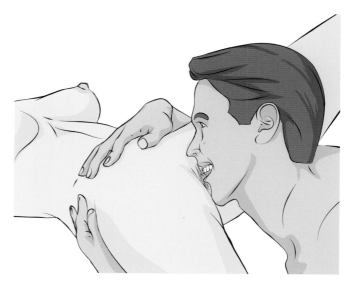

The Nibble

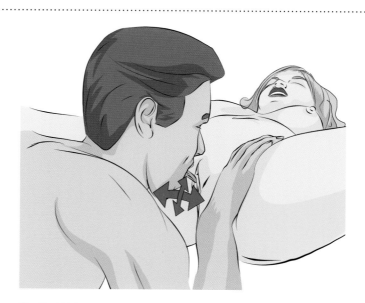

The Hard Lick

CHEAT SHEET: SPECIAL EXTRAS

When receiving oral sex, often a woman will need an extra sensation to send her over the edge of climax. Try any of these special extras as your tongue works its magic, and see if one helps tip the scale in your orgasm-inspiring favor.

- Reach up and pinch a nipple (or two).
- Grasp her breasts.
- Tickle the back of her knee or caress the backs of her thighs and calves.
- With one or both hands, squeeze and massage her butt cheeks.
- If your girl is into a little domination, hold her hands down by her sides (yes, she is your prisoner to devour).

12. THE CLIT SUCK: Once she's riding high, gently pull back her clitoral hood (if her clit isn't already exposed) and gently suck on her uncovered nub like you would a nipple. Add a flicking motion with your tongue and she just might shoot through the headboard.

13. THE HUMMER: Take her clit into your lips and softly hum, or make a sound like you're really enjoying what you're tasting—"Mmm." The sound of your voice and the tingling sensation of your vibrating lips on her nether parts is a heady combination.

14. UNEXPECTED SENSATIONS: Try sucking on ice or a mint, or use stimulating lubricants to add some extra sensations to your oral moves. (Please note: While it's fun to put things like whipped cream and chocolate on her body, keep sugary foods away from her vagina. Sugar can cause yeast infections, and that's no fun for either of you.)

Remember, if your girl seems to be really enjoying what you're doing, don't stop until she's gone over the top!

Hot Lickin' Positions

It may take a while for your lady to climax during your oral performance, so it would be wise to choose a comfortable position. And in some cases, the wow factor may be what you're after and could even speed up her reaction time. Here are a few of our favorite positions to get the licks done right. We've conveniently rated them out of five points in three categories: naughtiness, comfort, and creativity. You find the ones that work best for you and your girl.

1. LICKTIONARY

This is the oral counterpart for missionary position. She lies on her back, with her legs spread, you kneel, or lie stomach down before her honey hole. Change it up by having her draw her legs straight up toward the ceiling or resting them over your shoulders.

● ● ● ● ● COMFORT
● ● ● ● ● CREATIVITY
● ● ● ● ● NAUGHTINESS

2. BEND OVER BABY »

Have your lady bend over the back of the couch, the edge of the bed, or even reach down to touch her toes. You can also have her on all fours. The key is, you lick her from behind. This is a very naughty, sexy move that will have her panting for more.

● ● ● ● ● COMFORT
● ● ● ● ● CREATIVITY
● ● ● ● ● NAUGHTINESS

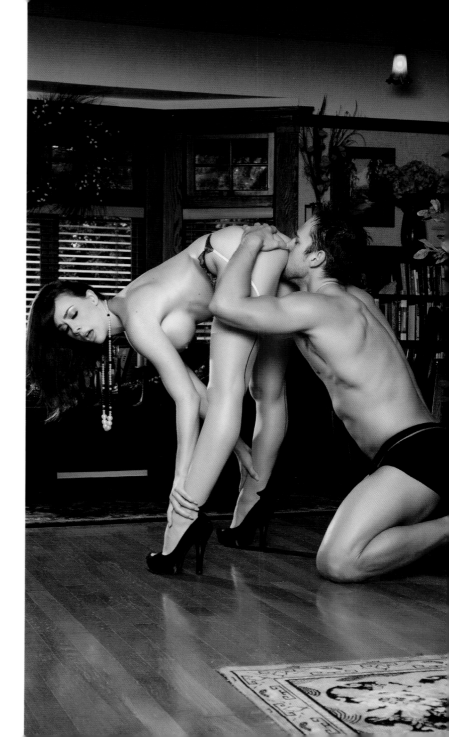

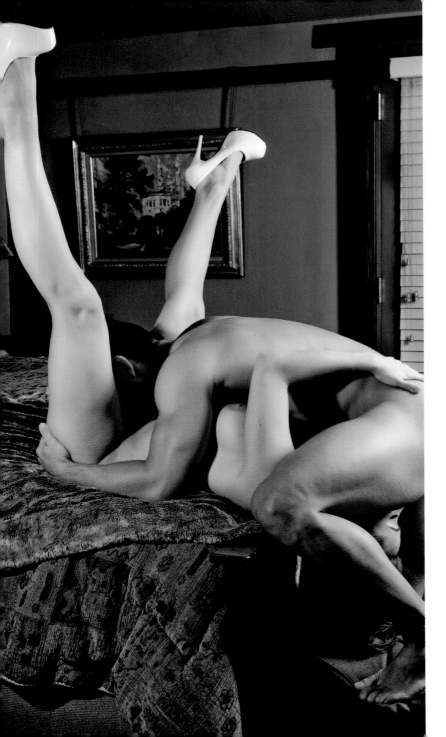

« 3. SIXTY-NINE (69)

This is our classic, naughty favorite. In this position, you simultaneously please each other orally. Sixty-nine has multiple subsets including her on top, him on top, side to side, and the more exotic seated upright, or standing positions. The upside is the mutual pleasure is ultra exciting, on the down side you may lose your rhythm or forget your goal of bringing her off first.

●—●—●—●—● COMFORT
●—●—●—●—● CREATIVITY
●—●—●—●—● NAUGHTINESS

4. JELLY SANDWICH

It's time to get really messy and let her sit on your face as you munch. She can straddle your face on her knees while you lie below her, or you can sit up and she can straddle you on her feet. Try it frontways, and back ways, any way you do it is going to be a deliciously naughty delight.

●—●—●—●—● COMFORT
●—●—●—●—● CREATIVITY
●—●—●—●—● NAUGHTINESS

5. CROSS SEXION »

Have her lie on her side with her bottom leg bent and her top leg open toward the ceiling. You lie perpendicular to her and nuzzle up into her crotch, resting your head on her thigh. Help her support her leg with your hand, or let her drape it over your head, or torso.

●——●——●——●——● COMFORT
●——●——●——●——● CREATIVITY
●——●——●——●——● NAUGHTINESS

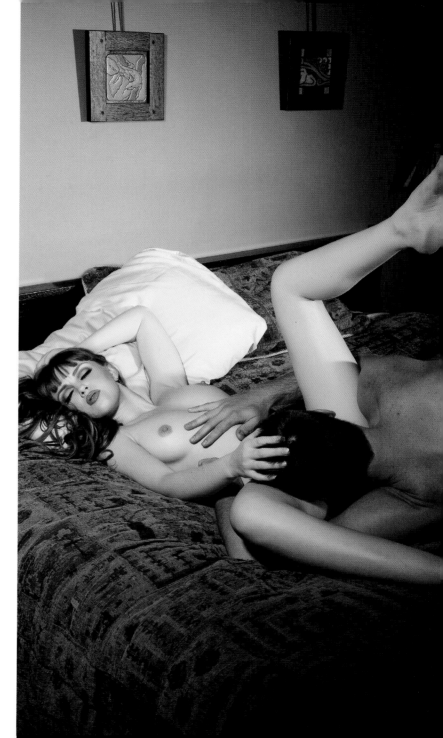

SEXtracurricular Activities: Find Her Favorite Technique

It's time to put your knowledge to practice. Here's the ultimate cunnilingus training exercise.

. . . .

1. WOO HER. Invite your favorite lady out on a nice date and enjoy a little bit of intimate time. It's important that she connect with you and that you give her an opportunity to relax and let go of the day's worries. Help her feel appreciated and beautiful *before* you slip her out of her thong. When the time is right, after a few kisses are shared, have her shed her clothes, but keep yours on. (You can take your shirt off, and even change into sweatpants if that's more comfortable, but don't let your eager penis out to play before its turn.)

2. COMPLIMENT HER. Tell her that this is all about her, that you want to make her feel good. Lavish her with praise, tell her how much you enjoy her body, and how much you want a taste of her.

3. CHOOSE A POSITION. Pick something that is comfortable enough for you to settle in to for as long as it takes.

4. PRACTICE MAKES PERFECT. Practice each of the techniques that you've learned in this chapter. Note which ones she responds to best. If you find one that really rocks her world, keep at it, keep at it, and don't you dare stop until she comes.

5. HAVE A HAPPY ENDING. After she's satiated, you can let your bulging anaconda out of your shorts. Chances are, she'll be eager to hop on top and rock her way to a second orgasm, taking you along for the ride this time.

Now that you've mastered the art of oral sex, be prepared for your partner to develop serious cravings to wrap her legs around your face! Enjoy the gratification that come from giving her pleasure. Says Al, a forty-something computer guru, "I enjoy giving oral sex more than receiving, and sometimes more than intercourse. Knowing that a woman is writhing around in pleasure because of my tongue is a big turn on, and I'm happy to give that pleasure to her."

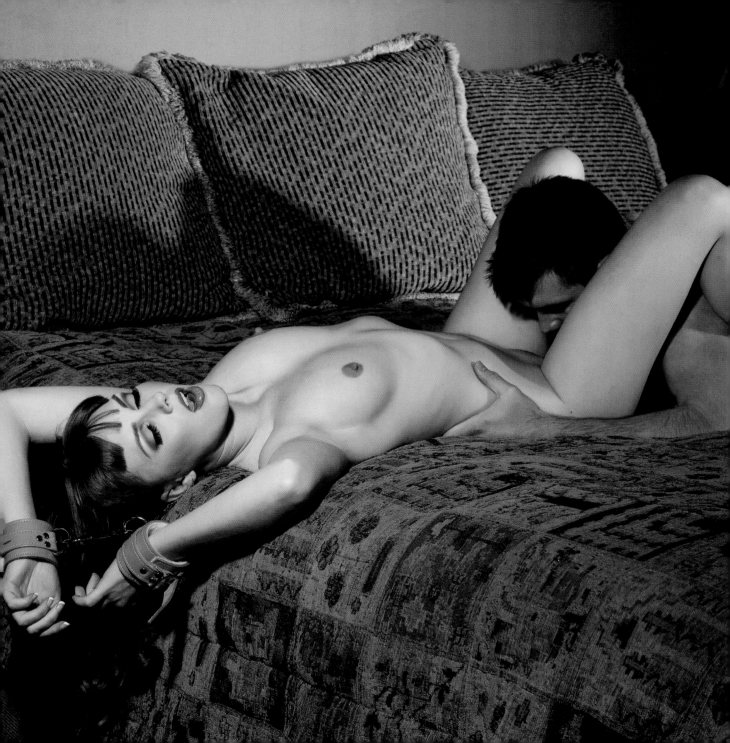

CHAPTER 5

Fun with Dick

Mastering the Bump 'n Grind

Her Jane does indeed love your Dick. While not all women experience orgasm via good, old-fashioned fucking, there's also nothing like quite like it. Being filled with your penis provides pleasurable pressure for her and great physical intimacy for the both of you. In this chapter, we'll discuss tips and techniques on how to properly apply your cock to her cunt, and how to get her screaming for more.

"LONG, PINK, AMAZING. IT'S DICK-A-LICIOUS!"

– SAMANTHA JONES, *SEX AND THE CITY*

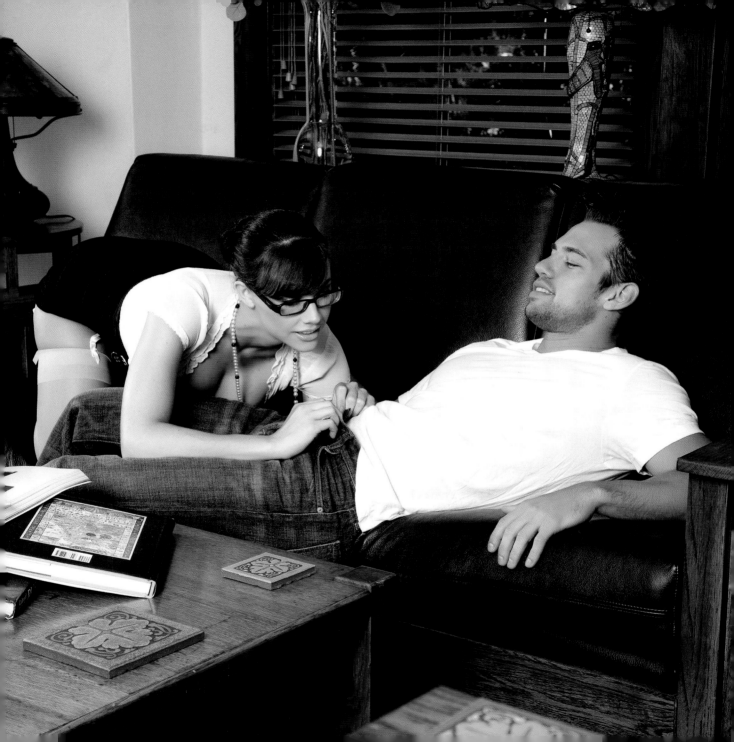

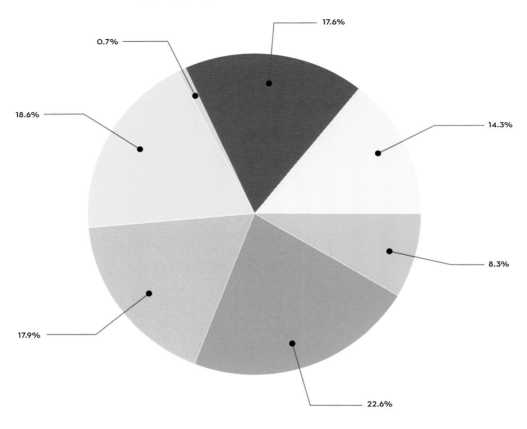

IN GENERAL, WHICH TYPE OF SEX POSITION BRINGS YOU TO ORGASM DURING INTERCOURSE?

17.6%

14.3%

0.7%

18.6%

8.3%

17.9%

22.6%

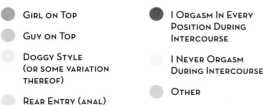

Girl on Top

Guy on Top

Doggy Style
(or some variation thereof)

Rear Entry (anal)

I Orgasm In Every Position During Intercourse

I Never Orgasm During Intercourse

Other

The slight majority of women (about 23 percent) orgasm during intercourse in girl-on-top positions. What's in the "Other" category? Many women specifically mentioned SPOONS, where you lie side by side, you behind her.

PENIS TEASE

Guys, penis-to-vulva contact doesn't always mean insertion. Just like fingers and tongue, you can use your tool to stroke and rub her clitoris. This can serve as a fabulous aperitif, or as the delicious main dish. An extra bonus for your boner: Her warmth and wetness feels amazing on the tip and shaft of your cock.

THE DICK TIP–CLIT TICKLE

There's something sexy about when a guy uses his cock to lightly tease and rub a girl's clit. Instead of immediately plunging into her, crawl in between her legs, give her one of your most devilish looks, grasp your cock in your hand, and rub the head against the upper side of her clitoris and along the inner lips. Draw it in circular motions around her clitoral glans, and when her hips start pressing toward you, try flicking the head of your cock up and down on her nub. As she becomes wetter, your cock head will slide easily across her vulva. Often, this type of stimulation can be even better than when you use a finger, because the head of your cock applies a softer pressure and can touch the most sensitive parts of her clitoris without causing discomfort. Women report being brought to orgasm this way, and many others confess that this kind of stimulation soon causes them to beg to be fucked. For extra fun, let her grasp your cock and direct the action for a while.

THE SUPER SHAFT RUB DOWN

Most women orgasm more easily from contact against their clitoris and vulva, rather than penetration inside the vagina—so why not use your shaft to rub those necessary spots directly? Line the shaft of your cock up along her pussy so that you can rub it up and down, back and forth, along her vulva. (Picture a hot dog lying in a bun, only much sexier!) To make it feel even better, try priming your cock with your favorite lube. It may take a little finesse on your part, but as you rock your hips, the stroke of your shaft against her most sensitive parts will feel exquisite—and for many women, it's specifically this type of stimulation that gets them off.

Try this type of dry humping (also known as *femoral intercourse*) in different positions. Most face-to-face positions work well for this move—for example, Book Ends, in which you both kneel, facing one another, and rub your naughty parts together. (The angle at which you spread your legs will adjust for any height differences between you.)

Gyrate Her G-spot

As we discussed in Chapter 1, the G-spot is the back of the clitoris. For some women, rubbing it just right with your penis can be an amazing way to come. Rowan, a forty-something writer sums it up best: "Please! Do not forget the G-spot. Please!"

Because the G-spot is made of erectile tissue, foreplay before your coital coreplay is a must. Kissing, licking, fondling, and caressing will cause her entire vulva to swell and her G-spot will become erect—all the better to stroke with your cock when you're both ready.

Once it's time for some good old-fashioned coitus, if you're blessed with a dick that curves slightly (or not-so-slightly) up and toward your six-pack, you'll be able to rub her the right way in Missionary position. For those of you who have straighter peckers (or dicks that curve in other ways), try adding a few of these into your repertoire:

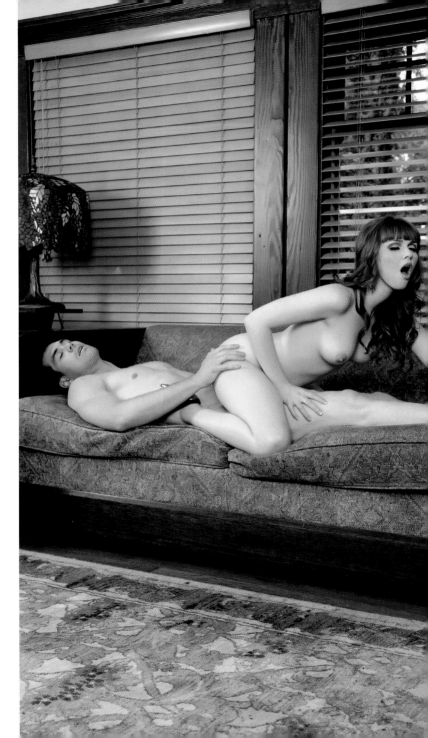

DOGGY STYLE

She assumes the doggy pose on her hands and knees, and you penetrate her from behind. Position yourself so that you're thrusting downward—the better to hit her special spot. She should arch her back and not rest her head on the bed.

« REVERSE COWGIRL

Lie on your back and have your lover straddle you, facing toward your feet. She can direct the speed and depth in this position, and best of all, she can direct the angle at which your cock rubs her inside. Have her lean forward and grab your shins or ankles. When the moans deepen, you'll both know you've discovered the perfect position.

DECK CHAIR (TOP RIGHT) AND FOLDED DECK CHAIR (RIGHT) »

These are similar to Missionary position. Stick your sexy self in between her legs when she's lying on her back and have her tilt her hips so that her legs are in the air. She can either hold them up in a 90-degree angle as you stroke her (Folded Deck Chair), or she can put her legs over your shoulders (Deck Chair). These positions give you the opportunity for deep penetration while at the same time providing a nice angle for some G-spot lovin'.

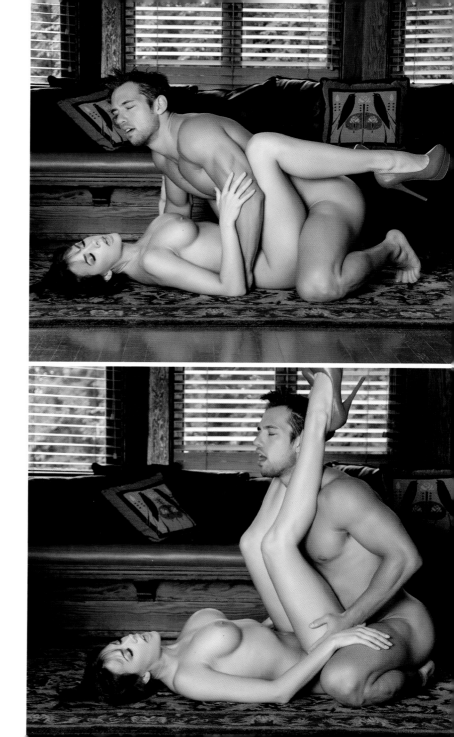

CHEAT SHEET: THE G-SPOT AND HER SEXUAL PEAK

According to Dr. Victoria Zdrok, author and contributor to AskMen.com, there is some evidence linking a woman's age with the intensity of her G-spot orgasms. The majority of women under thirty have higher estrogen levels, which causes their vaginal lining to be thicker than their over-thirty counterparts. The thicker vaginal lining cuts down on G-spot sensitivity. However, as a woman ages, the vaginal lining thins and that gorgeous G-spot is more accessible. Dr. Zdrok points out that this may be why women feel that they reach their sexual peaks after age thirty.[23]

LOVE ME TENDER

Variety is the spice of a good sex life, and there will definitely be times when she (and you) will crave a long, languid, slow fuck. When you take your time and go slow, it gives you both more of a chance to really feel which spots are the most sensitive to her, and there's nothing like a slow, sweet build to a singing, sizzling orgasm. Joshika, a thirty-seven-year-old mother and student, tells us that the number one most reliable way for her to come is for her lover "to kiss me passionately and to thrust deeply, slowly, and intensely." Here are a few positions that will provide gentle stroking and utmost intimacy.

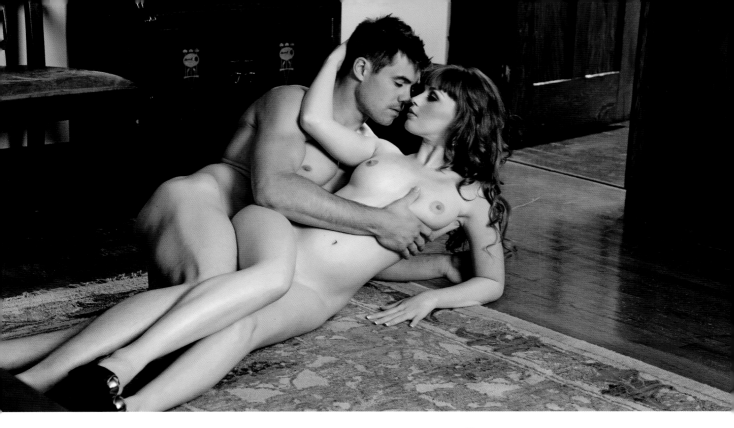

⌃ Spoons

Spooning is the one position most often linked with guaranteed orgasms. Have her lie on her side, and then snuggle up behind her. This position is excellent for intimacy because it takes less exertion, so you have more energy to hold her close to you, kiss her neck, whisper in her ear, caress her breasts, and/or pinch her nipples while you fuck her. She can lift her leg up for deeper penetration. She can also turn her head for some tender kissing or eye contact.

Fact or Fiction: Most Women Can Come from Coitus, or Vaginal Penetration, Alone

Many men and women are under the impression that a woman should be able to orgasm from vaginal penetration alone. Gentlemen, the notion that most women can come solely via coitus is, hands down, a myth. Twenty-seven percent of the women we surveyed reported being able to orgasm only from penile penetration, which leaves 73 percent who orgasm by other means. This statistic is backed by other research that has shown that about 75 percent of women report never reaching orgasm from penetration alone.[24] An interesting note: Even the beautiful and sexually iconic Marilyn Monroe never had an orgasm with any of her three husbands or long line of famous lovers. It wasn't until later in her life, when her therapist taught her to stimulate herself, that she could then, in turn, come with men.[25] Be sure to give your lover other sexy stimulation during penetrative sex by using your fingers, tongue, and toys on her clitoris. Following are a few good positions that are ideal for combining penetration and clitoral stimulation.

DOGGY STYLE

Have her get on the bed on all fours, and you kneel behind her. Your arms will be free to reach around and rub that cute little clit as you pound away.

STANDING MISSIONARY

Have her lie back on a surface, whether it's the bed or the kitchen table, so she's at the right height for you to stand between her legs and enter her. You won't have to lean on your arms as you stroke her with your cock, leaving your hands free to tend to her vulva with your dexterous digits.

ACROBAT »

This may take a bit of flexibility on her part. Get into it by lying on your back. She should straddle you, facing toward your feet, with her legs bent so that her weight is on her shins on either side of you. Have her lie back so that her back is against your chest. You'll have to take over the thrusting, and you can reach around and strum her clit.

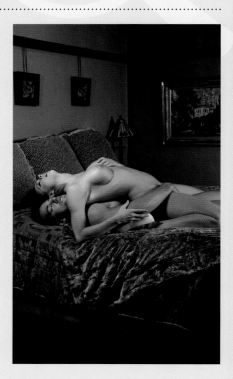

THE DELIGHT »

This is a face-to-face position where she sits on the edge of the bed and you kneel on the floor—or stand, depending on the height of your bed—in between her legs. She wraps her legs around you as you penetrate. This also works on the kitchen counter, a chair, the back of the couch—you get the picture. Guys, this provides excellent rubbing potential for her clit, and offers an intimacy similar to that in Missionary. Also, it's an easy position to maintain, so you can go as slow and long as you both like.

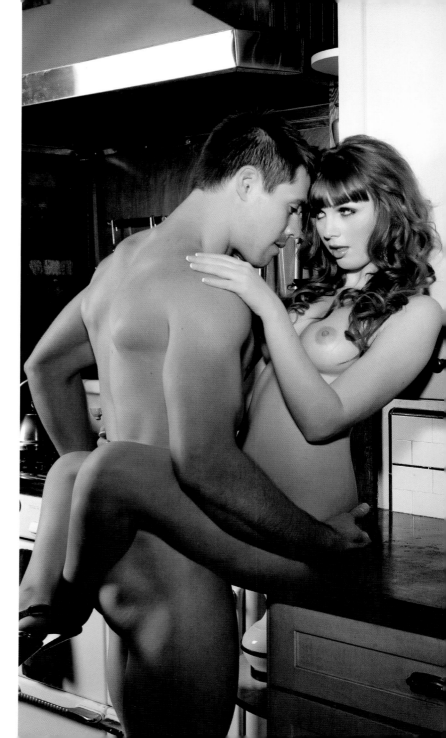

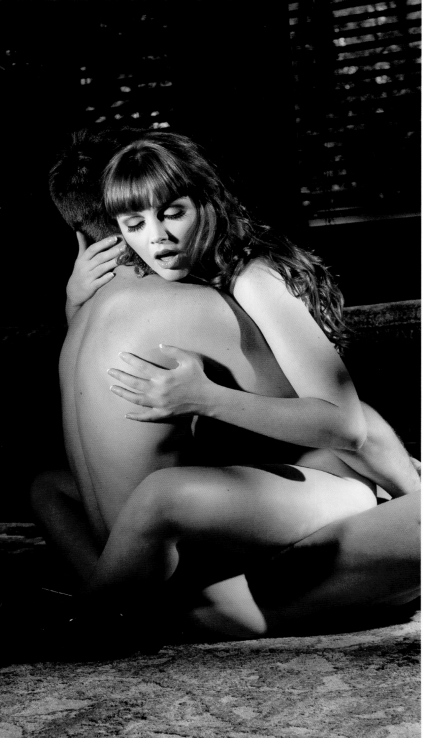

« Lotus

This position brings romance and pleasure to a whole new level. You sit cross-legged and she climbs into your lap and onto your cock, wrapping her legs and arms around you. Your torsos will be touching, and the motion comes from fluidly rocking back and forth together. You can also place your hands under her ass to guide her pussy back and forth on your dick. The intimacy of the embrace combined with vulva rubbing may soon have her moaning "Ohmmmmmm" in pleasure. Namaste!

Cheat Sheet: Keep Kinky with Kegels

....

Kegel exercises (first taught in 1948 by and named for gynecologist Dr. Arnold Kegel) are simple, yet important, exercises that work the pelvic floor muscle, or PC muscle. This muscle supports the bladder, bowel, and uterus, but it also intensifies a woman's orgasmic contractions. And a stronger pelvic floor muscle gives her more vaginal control—the better to squeeze your cock with and provide that sexy, tight feeling you love.

If your honey doesn't know how to squeeze her pelvic floor muscle, just barge in on her while she's peeing. She'll most likely stop, mid-flow, eyes wide and cheeks flushed in embarrassment. Just smile and tell her, "That's the muscle, baby!" *Note:* This is only a way for her to feel what muscle she should contract; she should not actually do her Kegels while urinating. Once she finds her PC muscle and learns how to contract it (without tightening her buttocks or thighs), have her follow this workout set (recommended by www.kegelexercisesforwomen.org).

1. Contract the muscle and hold for 3–5 seconds.
2. Release and relax for 3–5 seconds. (The relaxation period is actually just as important as the contraction.)
3. Repeat 10 times.
4. Do this routine three times per day.

The nice thing is, she can do these anywhere—while waiting in line at the (sex) store, or even enjoying a little morning coffee.

Once you've both practiced your Kegel exercises, you'll be able to add variety to your lovemaking. Instead of the old in-and-out motion, keep your bodies completely still while you both flex and contract your PC muscles. The feeling is incredibly intimate, sexy, and even orgasmic.

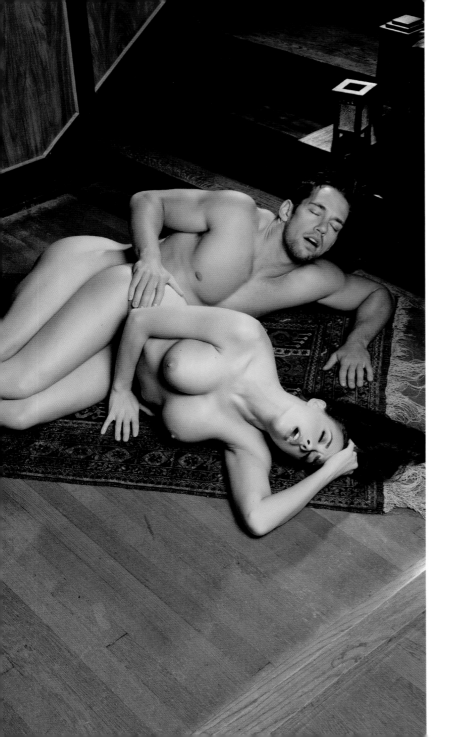

Fill 'Er Up

Sometimes, a girl wants a little tenderness, but other times, she just wants some good thrusting. Sally, a forty-four-year-old geologist, succinctly describes what gets her off best: "Fuck me hard." If your sex kitten is writhing and yelling, "More! More!" here are the go-to positions to maximize the size and feel of your cock inside her.

« Naughty Spoons

Get into the Spoons position and then transition easily into Naughty Spoons when she starts demanding more. Angle her torso forward so that her shoulders are at least a foot away from you, if not more. She should arch her back and push her ass toward you. Use your hands to grab her hips and thrust away! This specific angle gives great traction for intense penetration. There's also ample opportunity for a little hair pulling or spanking, if your princess is into that type of thing.

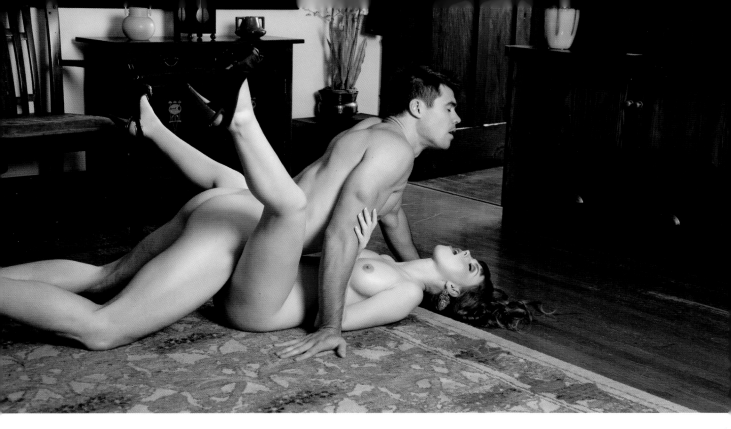

⌃ THE VICTORY POSITION

This is much like Missionary, but she'll turn her pelvis up slightly and straighten her legs out to either side of your body, forming a V around your torso. You can kneel over her so that her legs extend past your sides, or place your arms lower at her sides so that her legs rub your upper arms (she'll have to be more flexible for this). For a truly dominant stance, sit up slightly in a kneeling position and take her ankles or feet in your hands and spread her legs apart for her. The angle of her pelvis combined with the exposure and thrusting capacity in this position will make for intense penetration.

SEXtracurricular Activities:
Shallow vs. Deep (Thrusting, not Conversation)

....

We recommend experimenting when it comes to your thrusting techniques. Both shallow and deep thrusting have their benefits, and both can be exquisite during your next sex session.

The first few inches of the vaginal canal are the most sensitive and swell with blood when your lover is aroused. Shallow thrusting strokes the most sensitive part of her vagina and vulva and stimulates the edges of her clitoral organ, including the inner labia (see Chapter 1). To make it even better, shallow strokes stimulate the most sensitive part of your dick, the head and just below the head.

On the other hand, the inner two thirds of the vagina are sensitive to pressure, and many women enjoy feeling your cock deep inside as they approach climax. This is when deep thrusting is your friend. Also, deep thrusting brings your pubic bone into contact with her clitoris and vulva—and, with the right angle, friction, and pressure, can help bring her to orgasm.

Your assignment is to take two positions from this chapter to incorporate into your next sexual encounter, and then try shallow thrusting and deep thrusting during each, for at least three minutes apiece. You could try two similar positions, such as Deck Chair and Victory, or mix it up with two very different positions, such as Lotus and then Naughty Spoons. Talk to your lover, ask her which she likes and when, and pay attention to her physical reactions. She may like to start with certain stimulation, but needs something else for that nice finish. Who knows what you'll learn about your lover (and even yourself), and who knew learning could be so fun?

LOW-DOWN DOGGY (OR BASSETT HOUND)»

Doggy Style is a great position for intense thrusting action because the angles and access make your cock feel even bigger to her. If she's still howling for more, have her spread her legs as wide as she can and crouch down very low on her forearms. You can even press her shoulders and head to the bed. The lower she goes, the stronger your pounding will feel.

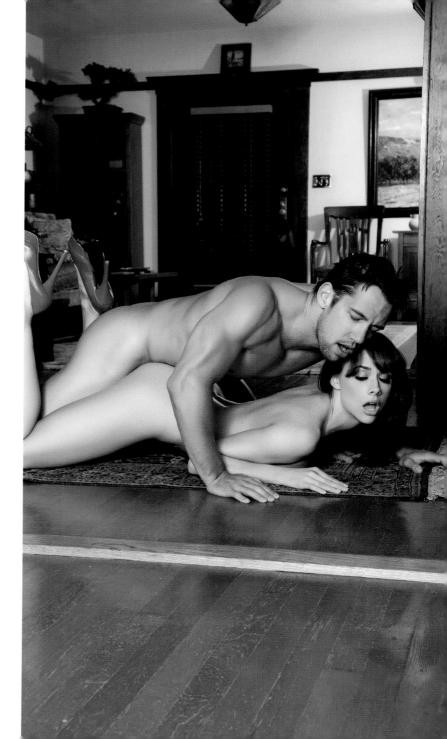

EXPERT TIP: USE A MIRROR

One simple way to inject some excitement into sex is to do it in front of a mirror, such as in the bathroom. It's exciting for her to be able to see your face, shoulders, and chest, as well as her own hot, swinging breasts in the reflection as you do it in Standing Doggy Style. If she's a little shy, maybe you both would prefer to zero in on the action rather than exposing the entirety of your bodies. Paul Joannides, author of *The Guide to Getting It On!*, recommends using a hand mirror.[26] She can use it to direct her own private viewing—positioning it as she likes to watch your ass and back in movement, or even some naughty in-and-out action.

PILE DRIVER »

You may have seen it in a porn vid or two. This is the perfect position if you want to add a little acrobatic fun to your sex life. Have her rest on her upper back and shoulders, with her arms braced under her hips for support. She will bend her body and bring her legs forward toward her head so that her ankles are on each side of her ears (or beyond). You stand over her, straddling her pelvis, and insert your cock into her. You'll control the speed and depth as you move up and down to penetrate her. This position is excellent if she supports her legs against a piece of furniture, like the bottom of a couch. This is another position that completely exposes her, so be sure to use your fingers for some nice clitoral stimulation as you drive into her. (*Note:* To avoid neck injury, she should not turn her neck right or left while in this position.)

Remember, when it comes to mastering the bump and grind, it's not only about what's on the inside (of her pussy, that is). It's important to keep her excited by stimulating her clitoris, vulva, G-spot, and, most important, her mind. Keep things fresh by trying new positions, techniques, and sensual actions to ensure she'll be coming back for more of your yum, yum lovin'.

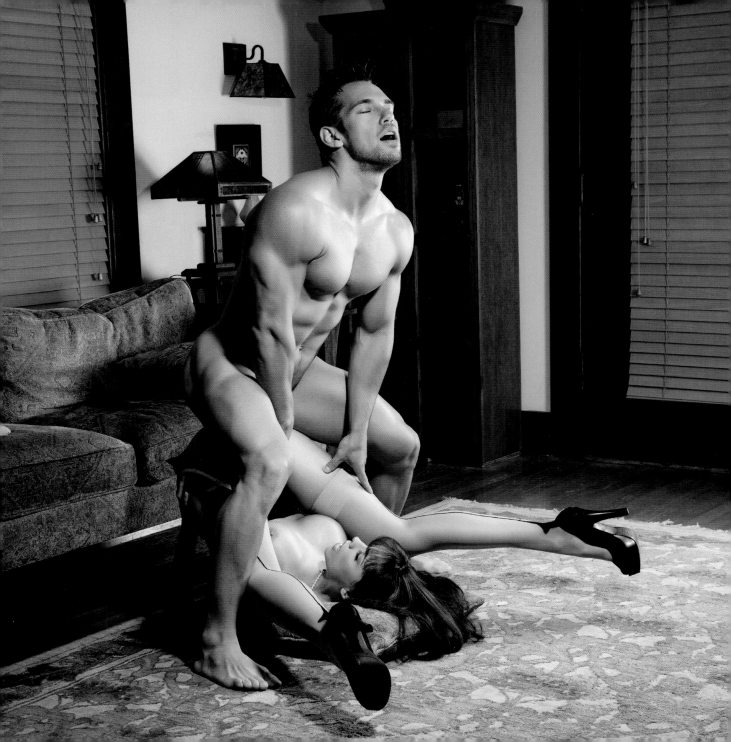

CHAPTER 6

AND ANAL

APPROACHING ASS-TASTIC AMUSEMENT

Mere inches from her vulva, just south from her fourchette and a short trek down the perineum highway, lies a part of your lover's anatomy that is loaded with nerve endings and just waiting to be invited to the sexual pleasure ball. It's wearing a pink party dress, all puckered up and ready to play. It can be gently touched, tickled, licked, pressed, probed, fingered, and fucked. That's right, gentlemen, we're talking about her asshole.

The anus is an important part of her sexual anatomy and (on both men and women) has one of the highest concentrations of nerve endings in the human body.[27] Moreover, in women, the anus is connected to the clitoral nerve network, so that when you stimulate it, you are indirectly stimulating her main sensory sex organ as well. [28]

"I WOULD LOVE TO SHOW UP BUT IT'S ACTUALLY ANAL SEX NIGHT AT THE GOLD HOUSE, SO...."

– ARI GOLD,
ENTOURAGE

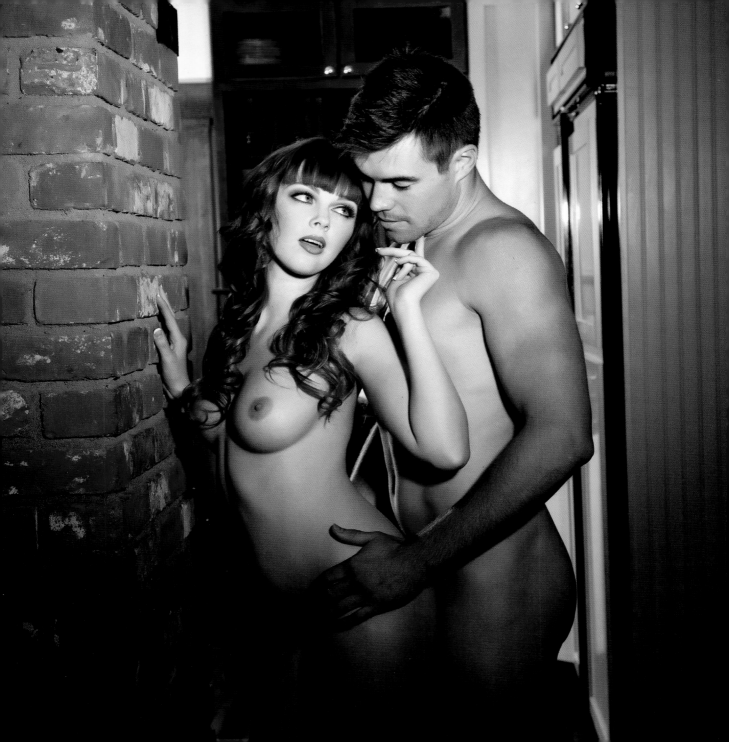

What Does She Really Think About Anal Play?

If you've dabbled in the art of anal stimulation, you are probably already aware that different women enjoy different types of touch in this über-sensitive area. There are some women who would prefer you to never go there, *ever*. For others, a gentle pressing on the outside of her rosebud during a languid oral sex session is the perfect amount of contact, and she'll never want anything more. Some women enjoy a little finger insertion or even a nice tongue tease. Other women absolutely love full-throttled anal sex (we're talking a good pounding with your cock here, guys), and a few women can achieve orgasm through this sex act alone.[29] More often than not, your lover will enjoy a variety of moves with anal play, depending on the sex act you're engaged in and her mood. The most important things to keep in mind are to always be loving with her little puckerhole, play to her (and your) comfort levels, and follow the code of safe anal conduct.

Cheat Sheet:
Women Disclose on Their Anal Experiences

As many as 5 to 10 percent of sexually active straight women engage in receptive anal intercourse (i.e., a penis inserted into the anus).[30] We surveyed women about their experiences with anal play and sex, including anal fingering, licking, and toy and cock penetration. Of the women we surveyed, 17 percent said they have been on the receiving end of anal sex play and loved it, while 24 percent have never done it and don't want to. Here are some of their comments:

"My husband is not too keen to touch the area.
He doesn't realize that it would seriously blow my mind."
—*Martha, 39, poetess*

"He just didn't know how to get it in there without hurting me,
so we gave up."
—*Nancy, 27, waitress*

"I come without any other stimulation, hard and very differently
than I do during vaginal sex. Uncontrollable spasms overwhelm me.
I feel like an animal and sound somewhat like one, too."
—*Kaytie, 45, stylist*

"A well-timed finger insertion can add to clitoral stimulation,
or a tongue caressing the area around the anus can be a heavenly
sensation, but no dicks up there please!"
—*Lily, 33, herbalist*

"Second best orgasm of my life was me on top, Cowgirl, but with him in my ass...
Something about my empty, wanting cunt rubbing on his stomach."
—*Tonya, 52, sex educator*

Analatomy

Understanding the anatomy of the anus is the first step in knowing how to bring her pleasure. Let's take a quick walk over the terrain of her tush in order to better empower you as a lover.

Her Anus

Also called the anal canal and less than an inch (2.5 centimeters) long, her little puckerhole is the guardian to the rectum, the visible little nubbin you can touch and tickle and tantalize to your heart's delight (provided she's comfortable with that). In addition to all of the nerve endings, the anal canal has two sphincter muscles that sit right on top of one another. (Think of them as two concentric rings in a bull's-eye.) The outer sphincter muscle is voluntarily controlled and the one she uses consciously to go number two. (Everybody poops!) The internal sphincter muscle moves involuntarily; this is the one that tightens up in response to unwanted intrusion and can cause her pain.

Her Rectum

If you have her permission and the desire, tenderly pushing into her anus will lead you to the rectum, which is between 5 and 9 inches (12.7 and 22.8 centimeters) long. Gently angling a finger toward the front of her body while in this passageway can indirectly stimulate the perineal sponge and G-spot. A special note on both the anus and rectum: These are only passageways, not storage areas, for feces, so you will only encounter trace amounts of poo, if any.[31] (We'll address hygiene concerns shortly.)

If you plan on inserting anything into her butt that is longer than about 3 inches (7.6 centimeters), you should know that her rectum curves and tilts. The lower rectum tilts toward the front of her body for approximately 3 inches (7.6 centimeters), then curves back toward the spine for a few inches, and then tilts slightly forward again to meet with the colon.[32] If you are inserting a long finger, toy, or your cock into her, gently navigate her passageways so that you don't miss any of the soft bends and cause undue pain.

Her Colon

Moving through the rectum will lead you to the sigmoid, or pelvic, colon. If you insert anything longer than approximately 9 inches (22.8 centimeters), you will encounter the colon, and this is indeed a storage area for poo. The typical anal aficionado does not usually have to worry about entering the colon, as this area is reserved for seriously large toys and anal fisters. If you are both interested in taking your anal explorations in these directions, we recommend reading *Ultimate Guide to Anal Sex, 2nd Edition* (Cleis Press), by Tristan Taormino.

Rules of Engagement (or Your Code for Anal Conduct)

When it comes to anal play and penetration, there is a set of rules and guidelines that must be followed for both safety and health. We understand that these guidelines may look long and tedious, but it's important to understand all of the risks associated with anal play, so that you and your lover can enjoy the lovely erotic wonders her butthole has to offer while steering clear of the potential hazards. Basically, the two most important things to keep in mind are that anal/rectal tissue is thin and more prone to tearing, and the anus is full of bacteria.[33] The thinner tissue puts both partners at a higher risk for transmitting STDs. And even if both partners are completely disease free, the presence of bacteria requires awareness and care to avoid the risk of spreading bacterial infection.

1. Get clean together. Take a shower and soap it up, guys. That includes her butthole, your hands, etc. You know the drill.

2. ALWAYS use lube!

3. BE GENTLE when you penetrate *and* when you withdraw. The set of sphincters are not valves; pain and damage can occur from friction in either direction.

Expert Tip: Which Lube Should You Use?

When it comes to anal play and penetration, Cathy Winks and Anne Semans highly recommend using a thicker, water-based lubricant, such as Embrace or K-Y Jelly. They warn that while oil-based lubes don't dry up the way water-based lubes do, the oil breaks down latex, which poses serious risks if you're using condoms.

Also, Winks and Semans highly recommend steering clear of lubricants marked "anal lubes," because these usually have desensitizing ingredients, such as lidocaine or benzocaine, which will anesthetize anal pain. The problem? Anal pain indicates you're doing something wrong and is the only warning sign you and your lover have to tell you that you need to back off, go more slowly, and use more lube![34]

4. Clip and file fingernails, and make sure any toys used in the butt are smooth and free of sharp points and ridges.

5. NEVER ever put a finger, toy, or penis that has been in an asshole into a pussy without first cleaning it (or yourself) with hot, soapy water. The high level of bacteria can cause terrible infections.

6. Use a condom, even if you're in a monogamous, disease-free relationship. The bacteria in her rectum can enter your urethra and cause urinary tract infections, or even infections in the prostate.[35] Ouch!

Be aware that it is possible to get her pregnant during anal sex. It's called "splash conception," and this occurs when your semen drips down into her vulva and then enters her vagina and impregnates her. That baby batter of yours can be some tenacious stuff!

7. If you use anal toys or objects to penetrate her, make sure they have a flared base or a rope or string to hang on to. The rectum is not like the vagina; there is no back wall to stop the toy from being sucked up into the colon and intestine. If a toy does make it to the colon and gets stuck, it may not only mean a blush-inducing trip to the ER, but surgery as well.

8. Don't use the toys you put in her ass (or yours) as switch-hitters with mouth or pussy. Cross-contamination can cause nasty infections. Along the same lines, if you use cheap latex or jelly toys in her ass, put a condom on them, or only use them once. These toys can be porous, and therefore act as breeding grounds for infection-causing bacteria.

9. Serious injury from anal sex is not common, but the experts at WebMD warn that it can occur. Possible injuries include causing hemorrhoids, tearing of the anal canal or rectum, or, even more serious, a perforation of the colon.[36] This is why it's incredibly important to always back off if she ever experiences pain.

Cheat Sheet: Approaching an Array of Anal Activities

Now that you understand the basic anatomy of her undercarriage, and you've dutifully studied the code of conduct, you're probably eager for playtime! There is such a wide variety of fun, erotic things you can do with her anus. We'll cover a few of our favorites to get you started.

For the Anal Novice

The first step is to find out how your lover feels about you messing around back there. The easiest and best way to broach the subject is to just ask her. But if you're a bit shy, try using a little anal touch as an accoutrement to your oral sex show.

When you're going down on your lover, slowly and softly use your forefinger to tickle the area surrounding her butthole. If she moans and opens her legs further, you have the go-ahead to lightly touch your finger directly to her anus. If she at all tenses up or squirms, remove your finger immediately. If she seems to enjoy it, simply leave your finger where it is and continue your mouth moves. Afterward, ask her if she enjoyed you touching her there and if she might like to go further. Congratulations! You've lovingly and gently opened the door to anal play.

"MY ANUS IS INCREDIBLY SENSITIVE. I PREFER FOR MY LOVER TO SIMPLY **PRESS HIS FINGER TO IT** AND DO NOTHING ELSE, [EXCEPT] KISSING MY THIGHS, BELLY, AND VULVA. WHEN HE'S GOING DOWN ON ME, JUST A TOUCH RIGHT THERE WILL BRING ME TO CLIMAX."

—KELLY, 44, PROJECT MANAGER

LET YOUR FINGERS DO THE WALKING

Now for some good old-fashioned finger-fucking action.

Now don't be shy, boys: The best way to know what to do to your lover is to play around on yourself first. When you're in the shower, all sudsy and clean, try sticking a finger into your ass. You'll get a good feel of the speed and pressure you should use on your lover. Push your wet finger in and out of yourself. Go slowly, and pay attention to the sensations that the movement inspires, both on the in-stroke and the pull-out. This shouldn't hurt, so if you're causing yourself pain, back off. And of course, treat her little butthole with the same kindness and sensitivity.

Now that you're armed with a little personal knowledge, take your freaky (clean) finger to the bedroom! Slather your finger and the opening of her anus with plenty of quality lube and insert.

Fingering her anus will be different than fingering her cunt. Here are a few techniques to try.

1. THE STANDSTILL: Simply insert one finger into her, up to your middle knuckle. Leave it there as you stimulate other body parts (e.g., kissing, rubbing her clit with another finger, licking her nipples).

2. MR. FRIENDLY: If she asks for some movement, softly rock that finger back and forth inside her, or move in subtle circular movements. This will stimulate the nerve endings surrounding her anus, as well as add to the pressure inside her.

3. IN-OUT ACTION: Just as you did to yourself in the shower, gently stroke your finger in and out of her anus. Remember to keep the same, soft pace on the in stroke and the out stroke. If she asks for more, you can add one finger at a time, gently stretching her open.

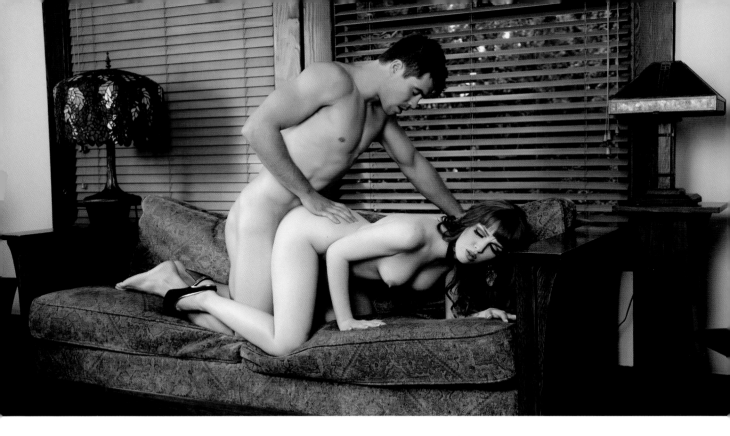

"THE MOST INTENSE ORGASMS I'VE EVER HAD WERE WITH **ANAL PENETRATION COMBINED WITH CLITORAL STIMULATION.** MY FAVORITE IS HAVING HIM EAT MY PUSSY WITH A FINGER (OR TWO) IN MY ASS. HEAVEN."

—SARAH, 35, TEACHER

4. HITCH A RIDE: Many women enjoy anal stimulation during sex. While you're doin' her Doggy Style, lube up a thumb and insert it into her anus. The added pressure can feel exquisite, and feeling your cock slide in and out of her through the tissue of her rectum might be an incredible turn-on for you as well!

The Original Butt-Fuck

The number of straight couples engaging in anal sex—that is, anal penetration with a penis—is on the rise. In 1988, the percentage of American women between the ages of twenty-five and thirty-nine who had experienced anal sex in the last year was 12 percent. According to the *National Survey of Sexual Health and Behavior*, published in October 2010 in the *Journal of Sexual Medicine*, that rate has risen to 21 percent.[37]

Women enjoy anal sex with your cock for the "full" and "stretching" feeling it provides. They also enjoy the perceived "taboo" nature of the act, and many enjoy doing it as a way to please their lovers. Some women will never experience orgasm this way, while others reach climax through anal fucking all the time. Just as with anything else, every woman is different. If you and your partner both enjoy finger pressing and finger fucking, you may choose to try penis-to-ass penetration. Be sure to follow the rules of engagement and enjoy!

"AS FOR HAVING ORGASMS DURING ANAL SEX…YES, YES, AND YES."

—BOBBIN, 38, INTERIOR DECORATOR

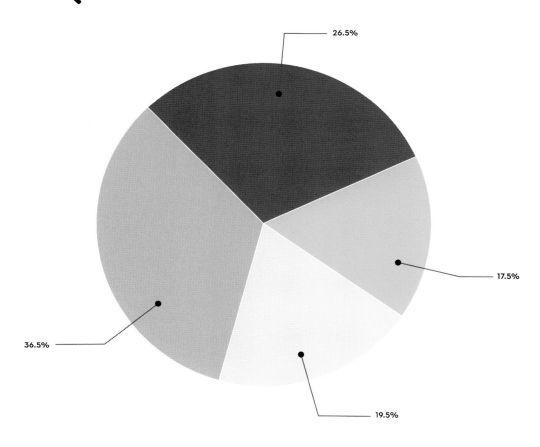

GUYS: HAVE YOU EVER PENETRATED YOUR PARTNER ANALLY?

26.5%

17.5%

36.5%

19.5%

○ YES, AND WE LOVE IT

○ YES, WE'VE EXPERIMENTED

● NO, BUT I WANT TO

○ NO, AND I NEVER WILL

Nineteen percent of men have given anal sex and loved it, while 17 percent have not and said they never will.

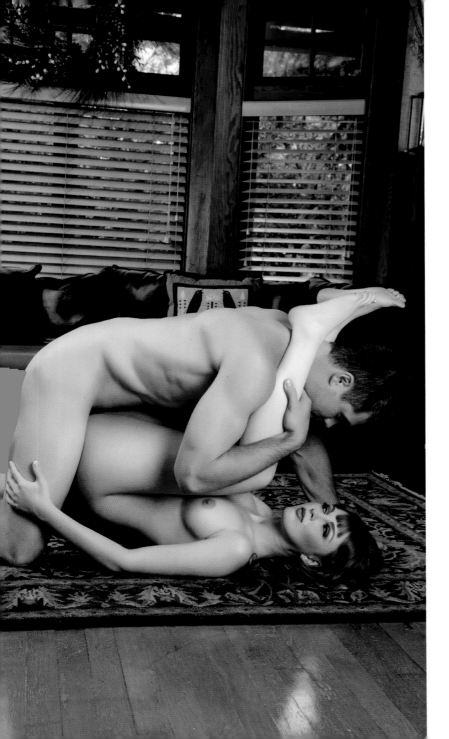

Butt-Lovin' Positions

Think of anal sex and most beginners think Doggy Style. However, almost any of the positions you use for vaginal coitus can be used for anal sex. Here are three different anal positions to try.

« 1. THE DRILL

This position is a variation of Missionary. Have her lie on her back, and you lie on top of her between her legs. She'll tilt her pelvis up, more than she would were you having vaginal sex, and wrap her legs around your torso or over your shoulders. If she can link her ankles together in this position, it may be easier for her to keep her pelvis tilted. Using plenty of lube, you simply insert your penis into her butthole, rather than her vagina. "I love anal sex in the Missionary position—there's never any pain in this position and I usually come because he can rub my clit at the same time," says Allison, a twenty-year-old pharmaceutical representative.

2. RODEO »

This is a great girl-on-top position to use for anal sex. You lie on your back with your legs together, and she'll straddle you, with your cock in her butt, facing your feet. Her weight will be on her shins and knees. A plus about all girl-on-top positions is that she can truly drive the pace and depth of penetration.

3. PILE DRIVER

Like its vaginal counterpart, this is an exotic position that lends itself well to anal sex. As described in Chapter 5, she will get onto her shoulders and upper back, resting her back and butt against the bed or sofa for additional support. You will straddle her exposed derriere and drop your cock into her. The thrusting action comes from you bending your legs—in essence, doing mini-squats.

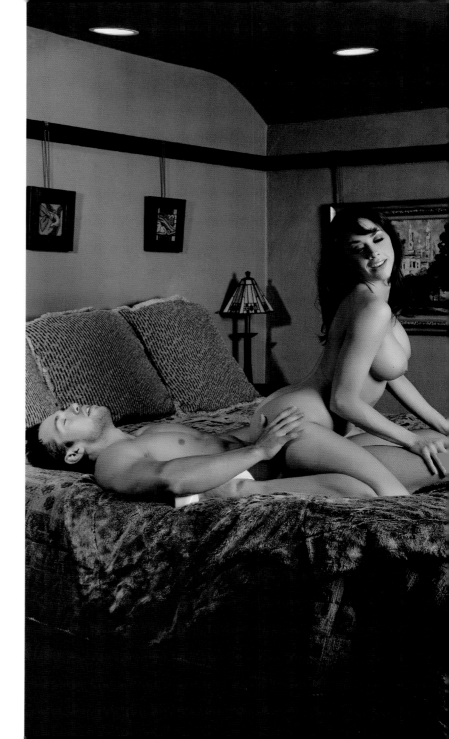

For the Anal Enthusiast: Rimming

If you're ready to take your anal play up a notch, you may want to experiment with rimming. That's right, boys, we're talking about licking her butthole. This is not for the squeamish or faint of heart. But for those of you comfortable enough to perform such an act, you may just send her shooting into the next galaxy. For many, there's just nothing like the feel of a tongue on the ass.

There is a risk of contracting intestinal parasites or a variety of STDs with this type of sex play, so to be safe, use plastic wrap or a dental dam. Those of you who have been with your partner for a couple of years most likely share the same anal flora,[38] but it is still wise to take every precaution.

If you'd like to try tickling your tongue against her derriere, take it to the shower. This is a nice way to enjoy foreplay together and ensure that she's as clean as a whistle. You can even use your own finger with a little nice-smelling soap to get her ready for your oral moves. Try lightly licking her rosebud as you reach up and fondle her breasts. You can also insert your tongue into her ass as you play with her clit. Chances are, she'll make it more than clear what she enjoys with gasps, moans, and exclamations of "Oh my God!" This is one act that leaves no room for vagaries.

As you can see, her puckering little butthole will make a fine partner at any sexual dance you want to attend. Just be sure to bring your favorite quality lube, clean hands, protection, the right toys, and a playful sense of adventure.

Peggy Wants to Peg

Pegging is the term used when your lover straps on her big ol' dildo and thrusts it into your awaiting anus (with just as much love and lube as you use with her, of course). Why, you wonder, would a woman enjoy this? First, it's one of the few sex acts during which a woman is penetrating you, which can be a huge turn-on for a woman, psychologically. Second, you will hopefully love the physical sensations it provides (and you may even orgasm through stimulation of your prostate), which is another huge turn-on for a woman. And third, there are all kinds of strap-ons and toys she can use on you that will also stimulate her clitoris and vulva. With this kind of toy, you can both thoroughly enjoy the act.

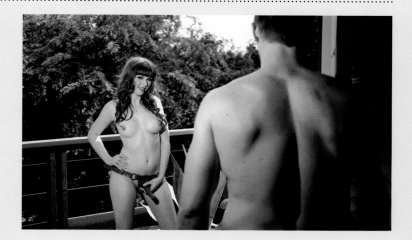

CHAPTER 7

HER OTHER BUTTONS

WHERE TO FIND THEM AND HOW TO PUSH THEM

Your woman is more than the sum of her naughty parts. Next time you are with your sexy somebody, don't just head straight to your favorite juicy bits (namely, her pussy). Try taking a tour of all of her other erogenous zones. Put on your explorer's cap, stick out your tongue, dip your fingers into some warmed up massage oil, and get to work licking, caressing, and playing with those other erogenous parts of her body.

"SEX IS DIRTY
ONLY WHEN IT'S
DONE RIGHT."

– WOODY ALLEN

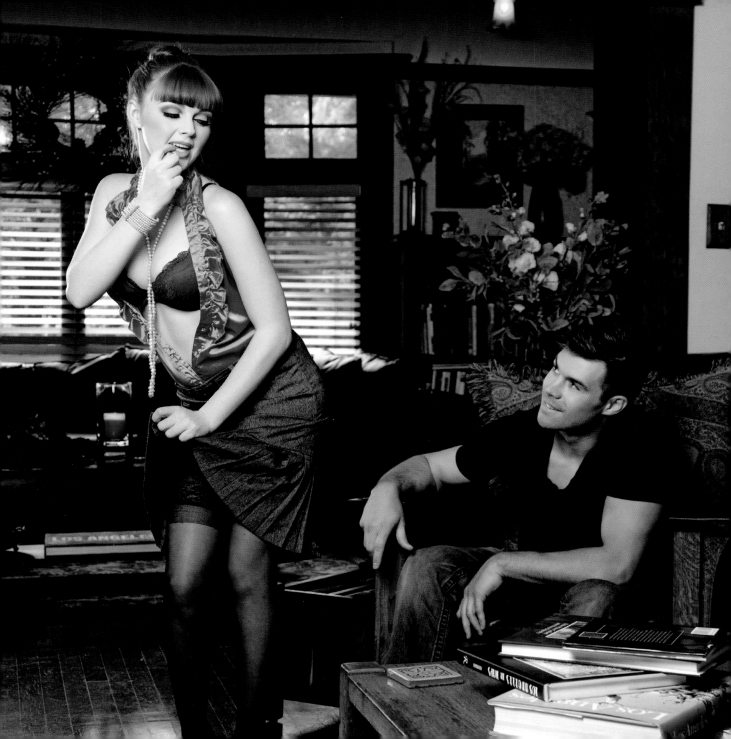

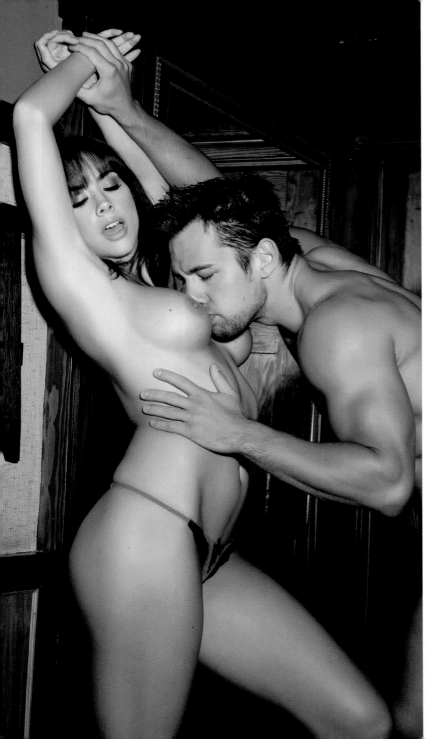

Hooray for Tits!

We're sure you're already quite well acquainted with those luscious scoops of flesh topped with cherry peaks of delectable perfection. Whether they're the size of a pair of cantaloupes or they fit perfectly in your cupped palms, these playthings are the delight of men across the world. Here are five sexy techniques for her breasts that you can perfect.

1. THE HOT FLICK

Cup her breast with one hand and bring the nipple to your mouth. With a stiff tongue, lap at the peak of her nipple using gentle and repetitive flicks. Then open your mouth wide and let out a warm exhale of breath. Repeat.

« 2. THE SUCCULENT KISS

Gently spread her arms up and over her head. Use your lips and tongue to wetly kiss every spot on her right breast with an open mouth, but don't yet touch her nipple. Move to the left breast and do the same thing. Continue to lazily tease her until she's arching up into your mouth. The combination of your wet, sexy mouth and the slow building will really drive her wild.

3. YOU'RE UNDER A-BREAST!

While she's on top of you, open your mouth wide and have her dip her breasts into your mouth one at a time. Let her do all the dirty work; now that you are under a-breast, you are at her mercy.

4. BACK AND FORTH »

While she's on top of you, grab her breasts and hold them close together. If she's facing you, move your mouth back and forth between her two nipples. She's sure to enjoy this double action!

5. THE TITTY TUSSLE

When a woman is in the throes of ecstasy, she's more receptive to aggressive moves, such as breast grabbing/squeezing and nipple biting. As with all things, start slow and gentle and work your way up to see where her boundaries lie.

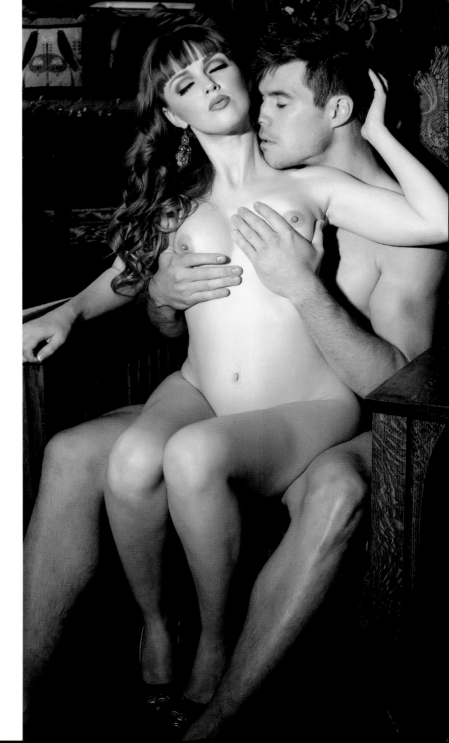

Cheat Sheet: Breast Esteem

In our survey, 71 percent of women reported that they like their breasts and 85 percent would never consider getting breast implants (which is good news for you guys, as only 1 percent of male respondents said they prefer silicone to flesh). We think this is a refreshing figure, considering all of the pop culture pressure for women to sport impossibly perky, yet large, bowling ball boobies at any cost. (We can think of better ways to spend our $8,000!) Remember to tell your lady today how much you adore her breasts. Yay, boobies!

Back to the Basics: Her Back

That beautiful expanse of skin that is her back is a treasure trove of sensuality, and an erotic back massage is a greatly appreciated act of affection. Treat your woman to one as soon as possible! Here are five tips to giving a great erotic back massage.

1. Set the mood. Turn the lights down low. Warm some sheets in the dryer and drape them over the bed. Play soft music in the background. Have your woman undress and lie between the warm sheets.

2. Start with her neck and shoulders and work your way down her spine and the surrounding muscles of her back using these strokes and techniques. The Glide: use your hand and forearms to create a never-ending gliding motion over the skin from the top of her body to the bottom. The Circle: with your thumbs side by side, locate knots in her muscles that need release and rub your thumbs in a circular motion, one going clockwise and the other counterclockwise, and then reverse. The Squeeze: squeeze the muscles between your fingers and thumbs in a kneading motion. The Scratch: scratch her back with your fingernails in long strokes, focusing on the length of her spine and then any areas that she asks you to touch.

3. Next, use those same strokes and techniques to massage her arms, hands, buttocks, thighs, calves, and feet.

4. Don't forget the power of your lips. Says twenty-something Michelle, "I like my partner to start kissing at the top of my spine and then kiss all the way down, blowing on my skin after his kisses makes me feel tingly and very aroused."

5. Some women have two especially sensitive spots right at the top of each ass cheek that can feel almost electrified if touched just right. Sally, a thirty-four-year-old accountant says, "Recently, a new lover was gently kissing my back and his lips brushed my lower back. I almost jumped off the bed with pleasure!" Brush your lips just above her buttocks to see if your lady has similar sensitive spots.

It's the Kiss that Counts

Any man worth his salt in the sack should know how to deliver a good kiss. After all, it's probably the first sexual move that the two of you will partake in. The first kiss is incredibly important to women. In fact, 66 percent of women in our survey said they would dump a guy after a bad first kiss.[39]

Follow her lead. You can learn a lot about what a girl likes by paying attention to how she does it herself. And don't be afraid to ask her! Consider the act of kissing a critical bonding agent for a happy and healthy relationship.

Three Awesome Kisses to Add to Your Arsenal

1. THE BREATHY TEASE KISS: Move in as if to kiss her, but instead of making full lip contact, gently brush her lips with yours before pulling back. Move in again, this time letting out a soft breath of air as you whisper by. Tease her until her eyes are closed and she's desperately reaching for you with tongue and lips before you give in and give her a lip-sizzling connection.

2. THE SPONTANEOUS, MID-CHORE KISS: At some point during the day, when you're both absorbed in mundane activities, find her, gently but firmly grasp the back of her neck, and give her a slow, sensual kiss. Whatever you do, don't take it any further than kissing. Simply break off the kiss, give her one of your sultry looks (or silly grins, whichever she prefers), and go back to whatever you were doing before.

3. THE "I LUST YOU SO MUCH I WANT TO EAT YOU" KISS: After a moment of your regular kissing routine, change it up a bit by gently grasping her bottom lip between your teeth. Try pulling her lip a little before releasing. Continue lip-to-lip contact, then a little nip. Always keep your bites light and playful (unless she says "Harder!" or bites you back with a vengeance).

Cheat Sheet: Kissing Rules!

From time to time, it's a good idea to brush up on your kissing technique and maybe learn a little something new. Here are our top seven tips for a knock-out kiss.

1. Start soft and gently touch your lips to hers. Kiss along her neck and jawline and return to her lips. No need to go in full bore with tongue and all just yet.

2. Once warmed up, probe her mouth with your tongue, but don't stick it straight down her throat. Some nice tip-of-the-tongue action is all most girls really want.

3. Women love whisker kisses! Treat your lady to a little five o'clock shadow from time to time or a nice brush of your beard.

4. Brush your teeth or suck on a mint before your make-out session.

5. Don't be too open-mouthed or too drooly.

6. But don't keep your lips closed and thin, either. You've got to give her a nice, soft landing point, so keep your lips puckered and pillowy.

7. Pull her into your kiss. Use your hands to keep her in contact with you by either wrapping them around her waist and ass or putting one paw around the nape of her neck and the other around her back.

Necking: It's Not Just for Teenagers

Remember those hot-and-heavy days in your rusty, old, hand-me-down Ford when you and your girlfriend left purple hickeys all over each other's necks? As an adult, you should probably forgo the neck marks, but that doesn't mean you should forget the sexy power of a little neck nookie. The rule of thumb for other erogenous zones on the body is that if there is a great number of hair follicles, there are more nerve endings as well.[40] The neck is a hot spot favored by nearly 90 percent of the women we surveyed.

1. KISS: Place gentle kisses up and down the sides of her neck from collarbone to jawline and up to the spot just behind her ear lobe. Says thirty-something Peggy, "I love the back of my neck kissed. It gives me tingles, goose bumps, and my knees go weak."

2. MASSAGE: With one hand, pull her hair up and away from her neck, and with the other gently squeeze and massage the back of her neck between your fingers and thumb. Even it out by switching hands.

3. BREATHE: Standing behind her, gently pull her hair up or to the side and, with your hands around her waist, exhale a hot breath onto the nape of her neck. Says Shelly, a thirty-something writer, "When my husband places breathy kisses on my neck, it both tickles and titillates me."

4. BITE: Once she is thoroughly aroused, start with gentle nibbles and, if she responds well, gradually increase the pressure of your bites. Don't chomp or suck too hard, or she may have to wear a turtleneck to work in the middle of July—either that, or explain her bruised neck to her coworkers.

SEXtracurricular Activities: The Art of Spanking!

Spankings can be a fun way to add pain and pleasure to your sex games. When aroused, your partner may enjoy the stinging sensation of your hand on her backside. Says Emily, a twenty-something veterinarian, "I like being spanked; the more aroused I am, the harder he can do it." Here are some tips for proper technique to ensure a playful and successful session.

1. Get her in position: over your knee, over the edge of the bed, or on all fours. When you are beginning, it's best for you to position yourself to the side of her body (rather than directly behind); this allows you to maneuver your hands correctly. As you improve your technique, you can also effectively deliver your loving swats during sex while behind her in Doggy Style or from beneath her while she is straddling you in Cowgirl.

2. Keep your hand relaxed. Your wrist should stay loose and flexible, as if you are playing a bongo drum. Smack your partner's butt using your four fingers, not your palm, and keep your thumb out of the way.

3. Alternatively, if your partner is sensitive but still looking for a spanking in your sex play, try cupping the palm of your hand and smacking her with the edges of your hand made by the cup. This gives a resounding spanking sound with less pain.

4. Consider investing in spanking implements, like a crop, paddle, or cane. Visit your local sex toy shop to try out the various devices on her bottom and select one that you are both comfortable with.

5. There is more than one place to spank a tush. Swat her on those round, fleshy globes, alternating between right and left, and then mix it up by swatting across both cheeks at once, right across the crack. If you want to add an extra zing, spank her sit spot—that spot where the upper thigh meets the butt cheek. Avoid smacking her coccyx (the very bottom of her spine just above the crack) or her kidneys (just above the butt cheeks in the lower back).

6. Between your swats, give her a reprieve by caressing her with your hands or laying down sweet and tender kisses. The alternation of pain and pleasure will drive her to ecstatic heights.

7. Watch the redness of her bottom. Depending on your intentions (playful sex games versus giving her a true BDSM punishment), if you see any welts but want to continue the spanking, you may want to distribute your smacks to other areas of her butt so that she won't have trouble sitting in her office chair tomorrow.

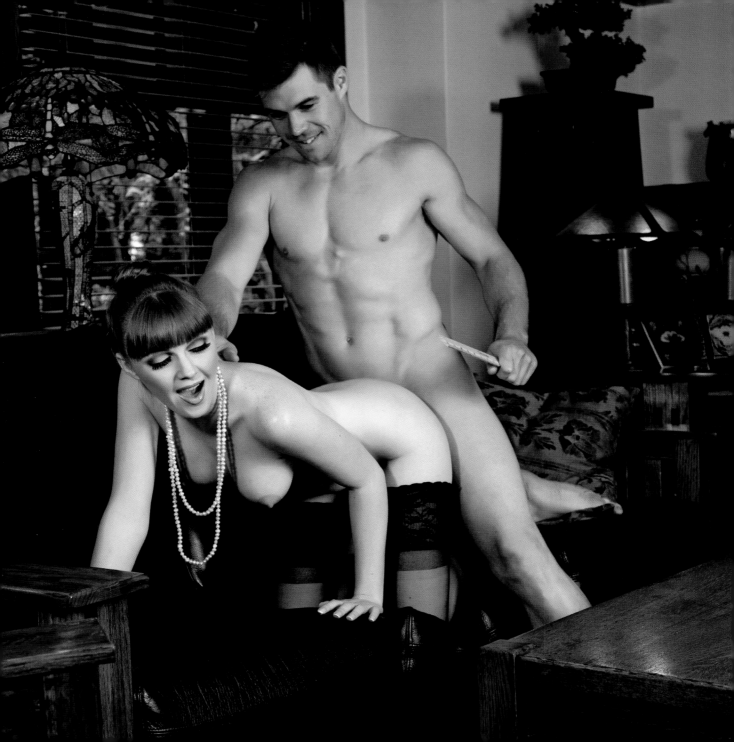

EXOTIC EROGENOUS AREAS

These locales are far off the beaten path. But just like a campsite at the end of an arduous backwoods hike or an authentic restaurant outside the confines of the tourist zone, the discovery of these secret spots can be particularly rewarding.

1. THE BACKS OF HER KNEES: These were mentioned as a favorite erogenous zone by quite a number of women. This tender flesh is a hot spot of nerve endings. While she's lying on her stomach, ever-so-gently stroke the skin back there with your fingertips. Or while she's on her back, draw her legs up skyward and lay some kisses to this delicate crevice.

2. HER INNER THIGHS: When preparing her for cunnilingus, tease her mercilessly by licking and massaging the sensitive flesh of her inner thighs. Take your tongue to the crease where her thigh meets the outside edge of her outer labia and lick all the way to the top of her leg and over to her hip bone. Travel across her lower pelvis just above her mons to the other hip bone and back down the crease at the top of her thigh, and finally down the opposite inner thigh. Repeat. Don't touch her pussy until she absolutely begs you to.

3. HER FACE: Try rubbing her temples with the tips of your fingers, and then stroke her cheeks from lips to hairline. Top it off with a few sweet kisses to her closed eyelids.

4. HER STOMACH: Give long, lingering kisses and gentle caresses—and even a few nibbles—to her stomach, especially to that area just below the belly button. Says thirty-something Olive, "My pussy clenches with anticipation if he kisses or caresses my tummy."

5. HER HAIR AND SCALP: Many women enjoy it when you run your fingers through their hair and give them a sensual scalp massage. Says twenty-something Talia, "A slow massage to my scalp is sometimes better than sex." Washing her hair in the bath or the shower is intimate, loving, and super-sexy. Says Clare, a thirty-something teacher, "My partner often washes my hair when we shower together, which I find very erotic." She might also enjoy a slight (or rough) hair pull during sex. Make sure you have the green light to touch her hair, though. Some women don't like hands on their locks.

6. HER EARS: Her ears are ultra sensitive to nibbles, strokes, and kisses on the outer edges and just inside. Some, but not all, women even like you to put a tongue in their ear. Says twenty-two-year-old Stephanie, "I love to have a guy put his tongue in my ear like he's French kissing it." However, other women find that slurping sound and wet feeling in the ear to be a big turn-off. Says thirty-seven-year-old Monica, "I love kisses on the earlobes, but keep the tongue out of my ear!" It'd be wise to find out which camp your woman is in before you dive in. And because her ears are directly connected to her brain, she will certainly enjoy the stimulation of sweet nothings or dirty words whispered just so. (For some tips on the art of dirty talk, read Chapter 9.)

7. HER ARMPITS: Nine percent of the women we surveyed said they enjoy a little stimulation of the armpits. Thirty-something Michelle says, "I once had a partner who loved to lick my armpits. It felt amazing, and very intimate." Many women find armpit stimulation ticklish instead of sensuous—in which case, it might be time to liven up your mattress with a whole lotta giggling fun. Laughter and sex both release stress-relieving endorphins and bring about a sense of well-being. So unleash the tickle monster!

8. HANDS AND FINGERS: In our survey, 24 percent of women reported they enjoy attention paid to their hands. Give her a hand massage and leave a romantic trail of kisses that go from the back of her hand and around to her palm and wrist. Says Kenni, a twenty-year-old student, "I absolutely love being kissed or bitten on the areas of my wrists directly below the palms of my hands." Some girls also get a kick out of you drawing her fingers into your mouth and giving them a sensual suck—it's the closest we'll ever get to knowing how it feels to get a blow job!

9. HER FEET AND TOES: Twenty-two percent of women said they enjoy attention paid to their feet. If your partner regularly gets pedicures or spends time painting her toenails, you might have one of these girls on your hands. For these women, nothing beats a sensual foot massage, and some may even be up for you sucking her toes (if you dare!). Says Chanti, a forty-something RN, "Toe sucking has got to be one of the hottest things anyone has ever done to me. My college boyfriend did it often. Sometimes we'd just be watching TV and he'd start sucking my toes. I could almost get off just from that alone."

10. HER NOSE: While a little Eskimo kiss might be a sweet and romantic gesture, what we're really talking about here is her sensitive sense of smell. In *The Smell Report,* Kate Fox of the Social Issues Research Centre wrote, "On standard tests of smelling ability...women consistently score significantly higher than men." She reported that a woman's sense of smell is 10,000 times stronger when she is ovulating—the better to smell your pheromones with, my dear.[41] Play to your partner's keen sense of smell by wearing her favorite cologne or aftershave and letting her sleep in your slightly worn T-shirts.

Most women love to be touched *all over.* Don't reserve all of your affections for her pussy, even if that is your favorite part of her sexy bod. Says Amanda, a twenty-four-year-old interpreter, "My husband says I'm like a cat, and I like to be petted. I enjoy foreplay and sex with as much body contact as possible. If there's any kind of contact between us, like feet under the table, or elbows on the armrest at the movies... Mmm. Good stuff happens."

CHAPTER 8

OH BOY, LET'S TALK TOYS!

ADD THEM TO YOUR REPERTOIRE FOR HER ENDLESS AMUSEMENT, AND YOURS

Gentlemen, sex toys are not made solely for her solo time! They can truly be your allies in the bedroom. Ten percent of women reported that using sex toys in bed is their most reliable way to achieve orgasm with a partner. Fifty-something Anne asks the important question: "Doesn't everyone have a toy box in their nightstand?" To become a true clit-ologist, you would be wise to learn how to use sex toys in conjunction with your own fabulous body to give your partner complete satisfaction.

In our survey, vibrators, dildos, and anal toys top the list of items that women love to bed down with. Says Peggy, a thirty-something office clerk, "If I'm burning stress, I go to the porn and usually get off in about five minutes. If it's more of a luxury kind of wank-off, I break out the toys and my favorite dirty book, then usually let my imagination take over."

> "THERE ARE A NUMBER OF MECHANICAL DEVICES WHICH INCREASE SEXUAL AROUSAL, PARTICULARLY IN WOMEN. CHIEF AMONG THEM IS THE MERCEDEZ-BENZ 380SL CONVERTIBLE."
>
> – P.J. O'ROURKE

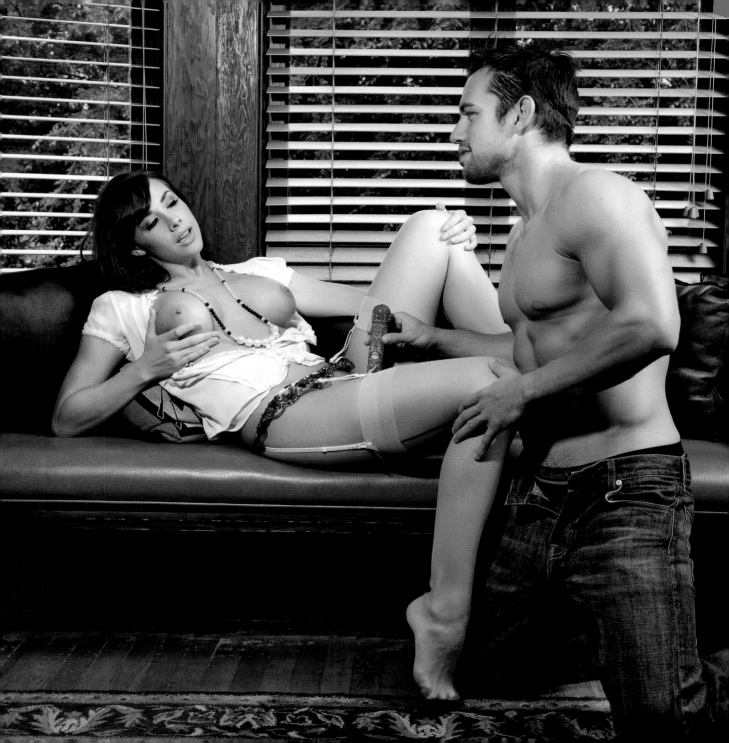

Expert Tip: Boys, Don't Be Jealous of Her Toys!

Says Jim, a thirty-something banker, "I don't like the idea of my wife using a sex toy. I should be more than enough man for her." Lauren Wolf, owner of Signature Sensuality (www.signaturesensuality.com), a couples-friendly sex-toy distributor based in Denver, Colorado, says that men should not be jealous of a lady's toy collection. "Sex toys are not 'replacements' and should not be viewed as such. They are additions and can very much add to your sexual experience without replacing anything or anyone. You might be surprised by how much your partner enjoys using the product on you or watching you use it on yourself, and vice versa."

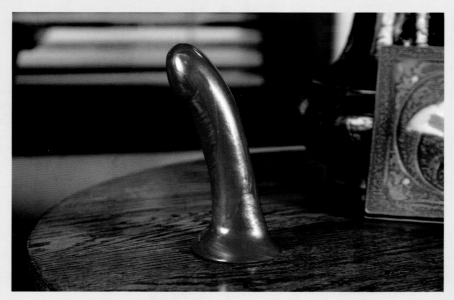

Dildo

WHICH AIDS DO YOU USE WHEN MASTURBATING?

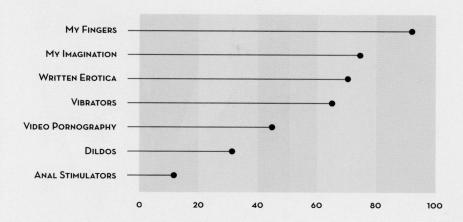

WHICH AIDS DO YOU USE DURING PARTNERED SEX?

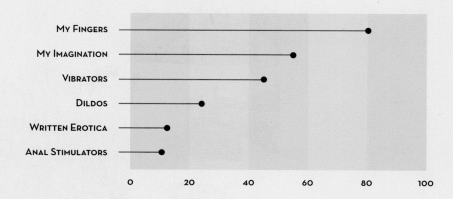

Dildos Are Delectable

Why would your partner ever need or want a dildo when you have the real deal right between your thighs? We can think of a few reasons and so can a lot of the women who we surveyed. Thirty-four percent of women admitted to using dildos while masturbating, and 24 percent said they use them during partner play. Dildos aren't only a way for your lady to "get some" when you're away on a business trip. They can also add some extra bang to your banging.

The Top Three Reasons to Add a Dildo to Your Partner Play

1. ADD A LITTLE EXTRA KINK TO YOUR SEX LIFE. Gentlemen, 54 percent of women tell us that they are interested in double penetration (DP) with a man plus a sex toy. (DP can be done with either both phalluses in her vagina, both in her anus, or one in her vagina and one in her anus—so be sure to ask your lovely lady what kind of naughtiness she's in the mood for.) Go that extra mile for your kinkstress and invest in a soft, fleshy dildo with a flared base so that you have something to hold on to. Also, choose one that is made of a soft, pliable material so that it has some give, which makes DP easier and less likely to hurt. Start with a smaller model, and graduate to larger models if your partner wants to push her boundaries and find that ultimate stretch. Remember to always use lube!

2. HAVE A CONVENIENT BACK-UP. What if your all-natural, built-in model is temporarily not working so well due to premature ejaculation or a case of whiskey dick? This is the perfect time to call in for a some back-up. There is no reason to make a big deal about a misbehaving hard-on when you can pleasure your partner with her favorite fake friend. And who knows, perhaps the kinky spirit will—um—inspire you to get back in the game.

3. EXTEND PLAY TIME. Dildos can provide a great way to add some time to your sex session, get her extra excited, and encourage her to achieve multiple orgasms by penetrating her with a toy before you penetrate her with your cock. Alternatively, use a dildo to play an extra kinky game by doing a virtual partner swap, switching between her plaything and yours. Have a clean towel nearby to put the dildo on in between turns so that you don't accidentally get it dirty by setting it down in dog fur or other household germs.

Diddle Her with a Dildo

Here are a few tips and techniques on how to use a dildo with your lover.

1. Always use plenty of lube! Even if she's naturally wet, toys seem to suck up her love juices more quickly than your cock will. Silicone-based lubes will damage silicone or cyberskin dildos, so use a water-based lubricant or put a condom on your toy.

2. You can maneuver positions using your dildo that are more difficult to accomplish with your penis. For example, if she wants to be fucked standing up but you're too tall to penetrate her comfortably, you can use your dildo instead. Or if she loves the feel of your cock in her mouth, but also wants to have penetration, you can accommodate her by stroking her cunt with the dildo while she goes to town on you.

3. Similarly, you can maneuver angles using your dildo that are more difficult to accomplish with your penis. For example, unless you have a penis that naturally curves up, Missionary might be a difficult position in which to stroke her G-spot. Dildo to the rescue! Have her lie back and relax, and use the dildo to slide in and out over her sensitive spot.

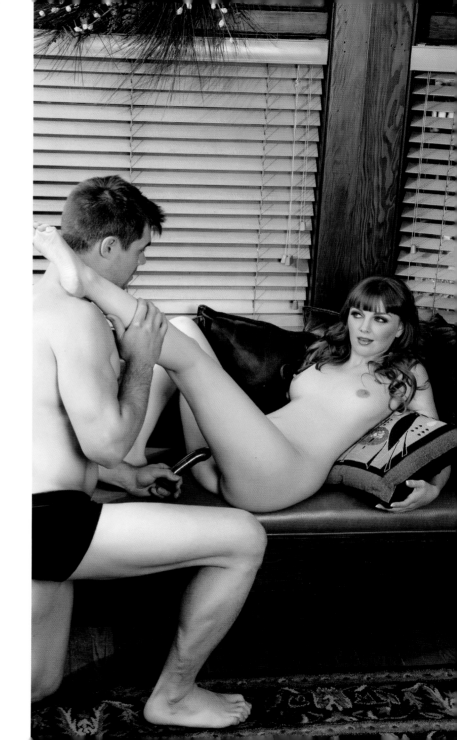

Cheat Sheet: History of the Vibrator

The first vibrator was a large contraption created by Dr. Joseph Mortimer Granville in the 1880s. It was originally installed in doctors' offices as a medical device whose purpose was to treat women suffering from muscle aches (same story with those Hitachi Magic Wands that they sell at Walmart). The device became popular with doctors as a way to quickly bring patients to orgasm—err, we mean *paroxysm*—rather than spending an hour for a manual pelvic massage (hey, time is money right?) as treatment for a condition called hysteria. Hysteria was a "medical" condition that was a catchall diagnosis given to women at a time when they were incredibly sexually and socially oppressed, and it had an array of symptoms, including "a tendency to cause trouble" and an "excessively moist vagina." (Today we call this condition *being horny*). In 1902, Hamilton Beach patented the first handheld, take-home vibrator, and, lucky us, the rest is history.[42]

Vibrators Are Divine

Vibrators are motorized sex toys that come in a variety of shapes and sizes, from phallic objects to small, egg-shaped devices to toys that could be mistaken for modern art. Signature Sensuality owner Wolf tells us, "Women are interested in what a product does *and* what it looks like. For a long time, the industry made products that were extremely phallic, oversized, and too realistic. Fake hair? Veins 'for her pleasure'? Simulated skin tones? Naked, airbrushed women with their hiney in the air—Really? I think most women prefer to shop for personal toys like they do clothing, accessories, and tech gadgets. We are attracted to shape, color, overall aesthetics, packaging, and, most of all, effectiveness!"

With these sexy new "for her" products on the market, it's no wonder that these battery-operated contraptions were reported as the most commonly used sex toy among our female respondents. In our survey, 66 percent of women reported that they use vibrators during masturbation, and 44 percent use them during partner play.

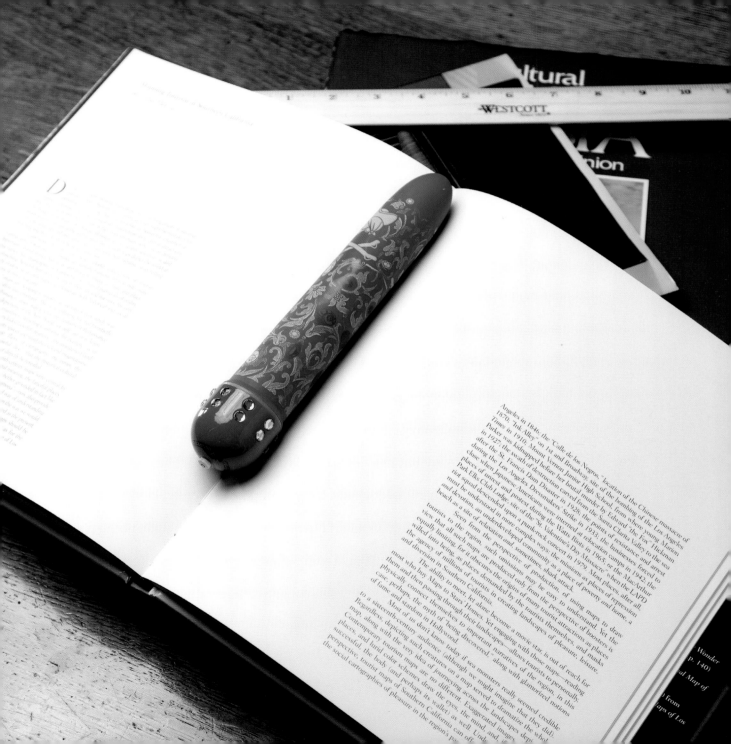

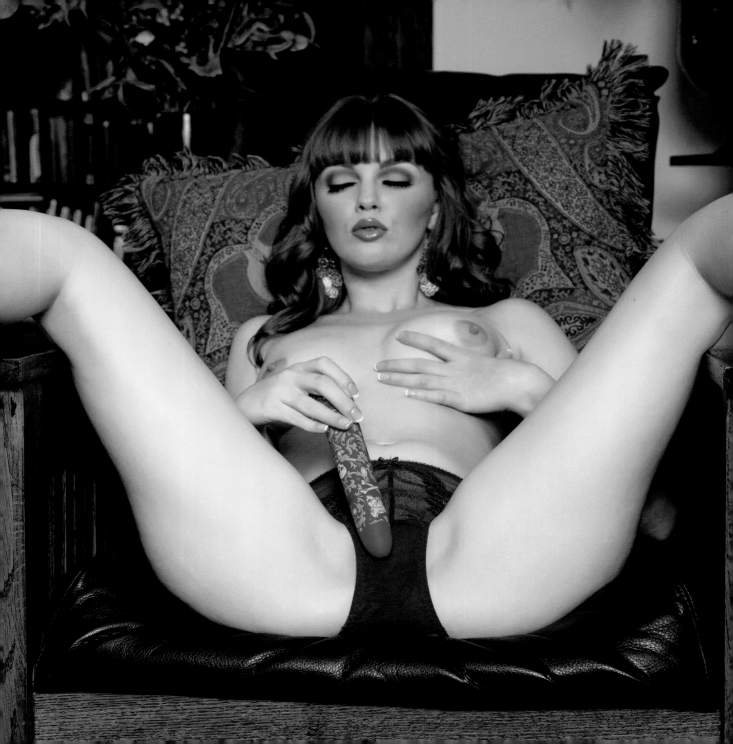

THE TOP THREE REASONS TO ADD A VIBE TO YOUR SEX PLAY

1. FAST-TRACK YOUR ORGASMS. A vibe to the clitoris usually ensures a knock-out orgasm for your partner. (If it worked for those naughty nineteenth-century doctors, it should work for you, too.) Interested in helping her become multi-orgasmic? Well then add a vibe to get a few bonus Os in. (Or at least one really good one!)

2. IT'S GOT THE RHYTHM. Do you have trouble keeping a steady rhythm? Often, to achieve orgasm, women, just like men, need a consistent pace. And sometimes your tongue or fingers just can't keep the tempo that she needs. Vibrators are great because they come with multiple settings from pulsating to escalating to a steady hum so you can choose a rhythm that suits her needs. Wolf says, "Why don't men vibrate? Sustained clitoral vibration is often cited as the biggest benefit toys can bring to women during intimate activities. The stimulation created by vibrating toys is unique and difficult to replicate."

3. BENEFIT FROM MUTUAL ENJOYMENT. Guess what? Vibrations don't only feel good on her. You can benefit from the sensations, too. After all, making whoopie is way more fun when both partners are in a sex-crazed state.

VIBE YOUR VIXEN

Here are a few tips on how to use a vibrator with your lover.

1. Just as with anything else, start out slow. Many vibrators come with different speeds and pulsing patterns. Start out on the lowest vibration speed and work your way up as she wishes.

2. Tease her. Lightly run the vibrator down her neck, over her collar bone, over her breasts, and around her nipples. Softly caress her inner thighs, letting the vibration warm her up. When she's good and relaxed, press the vibrator to the outside of her vaginal lips and along her perineum.

3. Once you have her gasping and squirming, spread her outer lips open and run the vibrator softly over the folds of her vulva. Lightly press the toy to her clitoris, remove it, then press it again. Ask her what she likes and whether she wants you to turn up the speed. Try inserting the vibrator into her vagina as you suck on her clit, or give her a slow finger fuck as you circle her vulva with the toy. Keep it playful, and enjoy!

Not Sure Which Vibe to Choose?

Here is a rundown of the fun toys that are available. Use them whenever you fancy to enhance playtime.

THE WE-VIBE »

The first vibrator billed as a couple's vibe (which puts the "we" in We-Vibe), this is a U-shaped vibrator that you hook onto her pussy so the bottom pad rests inside her on the roof of her vaginal canal (the location of the G-spot) and the top pad rests outside her body on the clitoris and vulva. It's made so that you can slide your penis inside and share the cozy canal while enjoying the good vibrations.

VIBRATING DILDO

This toy combines both the pleasures of the phallus and the pleasures of good vibrations.

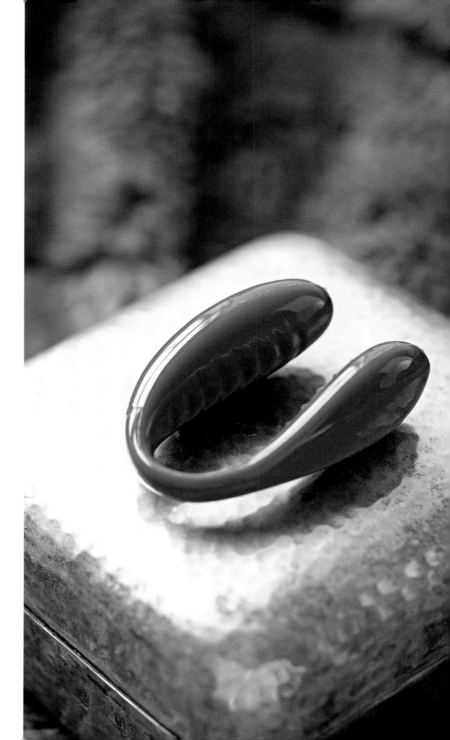

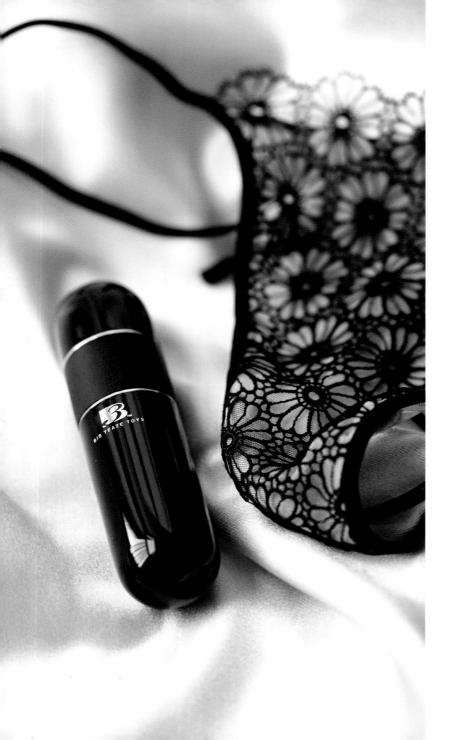

« BULLET VIBE

This is a versatile, egg-shaped vibrator that fits in the palm of your hand. The small size makes it easy for her to stimulate her clitoris while you attend to the rest of her, in nearly any sex position. Alternatively, you can use the bullet to stimulate her nipples, your scrotum, her perineum, or yours!

VIBRATING COCK RING

The cock ring offers the benefit of keeping you harder longer while the small vibrating attachment presses up against her clitoris. All aboard the sex-o-cock train to the land of Os!

REMOTE-CONTROL VIBRATING PANTIES »

These may not give you direct stimulation, but you'll get a whole lot of mental stimulation from delivering her pleasure via remote control. (Yeah, we know how much you guys like to have control of that remote!) She should wear the vibrating panty to a club, concert, or any other loud social setting. (A dinner table at a quiet restaurant might not be a good idea since the vibrations will be audible and there are only so many times that you can blame the buzzing on your cell phone.) When she's least expecting it, use the remote control to turn the bullet on and watch her face as she tries to hide her secret pleasure.

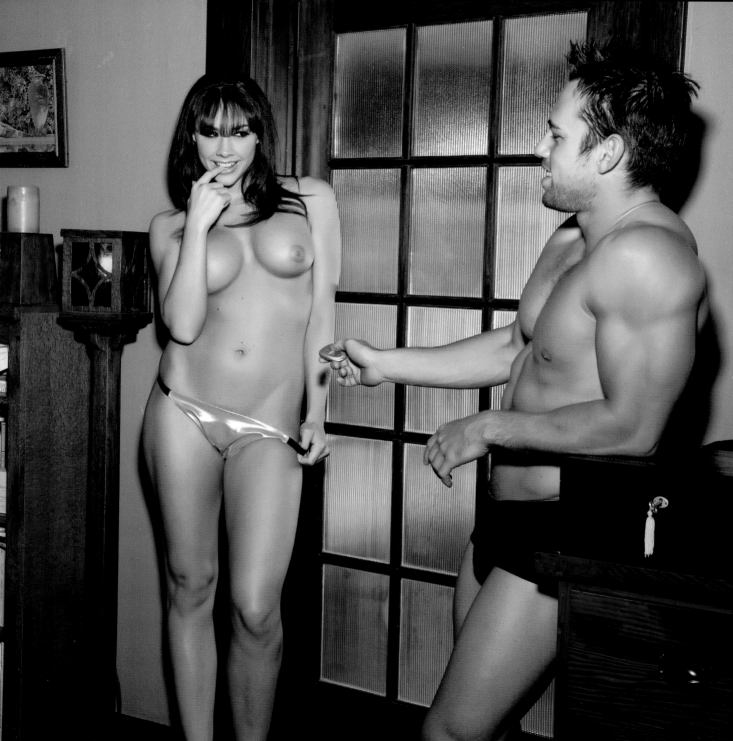

Anal Toys Are Awesome

If your chick is hip to the funky butt lovin', nothing beats an investment in some sexy anal stimulators. Anal toys include anal beads, massagers, vibrators, and butt plugs. Remember: Play only after getting her permission, and use lube! Read Chapter 6 for more information on anal sex.

Three Fun Anal Toys

1. ANAL BEADS, BABY

Anal beads are a sequence of round beads strung together on a cord or a stalk. Some variations have the beads increase in size, while others are all uniform in size. You can also opt for vibrating beads. During insertion, your partner will feel the pleasure of her anus being stretched and relaxed, stretched and relaxed as the beads enter her one by one. At orgasm, pull the beads out all at once for an added rush of sensation.

2. BUTT-PLUGS »

For a super-kinky public sex adventure where none will be the wiser, have your sexy lady insert a butt plug and then go out on a date with you. Watch her squirm with excitement as she sits beside you at the theater, feeling filled with promise. Every once in a while, lean toward her and tell her about all the naughty things you are going to do with her later. Give her enough teasing, and she won't be able to keep her hands off of you. During sex, a butt plug is a very nice tool to use to add that extra sizzle to your fireworks show. During your next Missionary session, reach down and insert that little bad boy into her ass. (Make sure it's lubed first, of course.) The naughty factor, combined with the anal stimulation, may just make her scream! You can also gently twist and turn a butt plug to stimulate all of those little nerve endings around her anus. Yum!

3. PONYTAILS

If your girl is loving the ass play, she's probably mischievous enough to enjoy a little all-in-good-fun humiliation game. Some butt plugs come equipped with floggers that look like horse tails. Next time you both agree your pony needs a little riding lesson, dress her up in her favorite negligee and insert the ponytail butt plug as the coup de grâce. Have her prance around for you, swishing her cute little behind, tail and all, this way and that. We'll let you decide when the show's over and it's time for a ride.

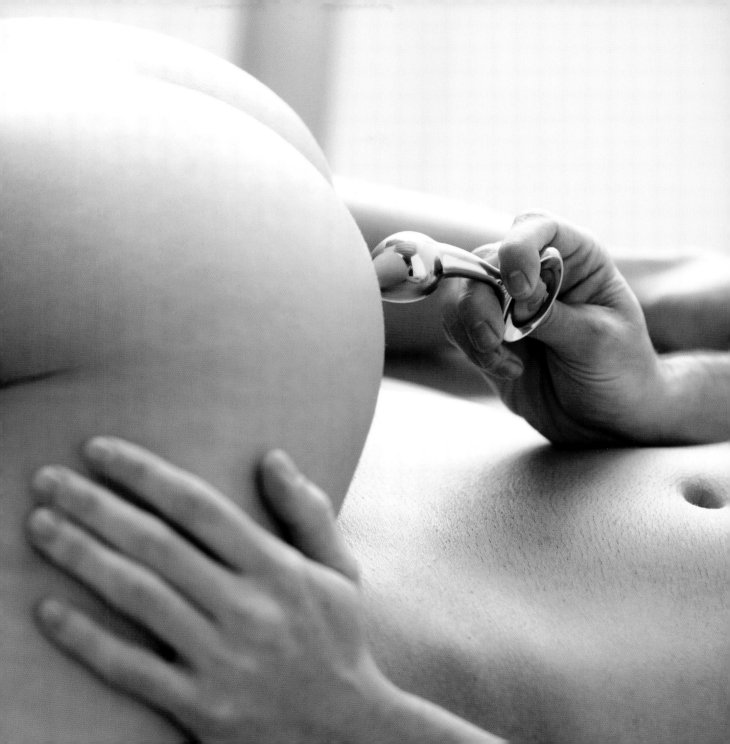

Ben Wa Balls: An Ancient Japanese Secret

Ben Wa balls were allegedly invented by a Japanese courtesan in about 500 AD and were said to be made of ivory, be coated in gold or silver, and contain a small ball of mercury that caused pleasant vibrations with movement.[43] Today, the marble-size balls are made of nearly everything except ivory, including metal, glass, and plastic. Ben Wa balls are inserted into her vagina, and she can then move them up and down using her internal muscles. Most women hold the balls in the lower 2 inches (5 centimeters) of the vagina, where they can roll back and forth over all of those nerve endings and the G-spot. Some come with strings attached for easier removal, others come as a free-floating pair. Not to worry: They can't get lost in the vagina (which is naturally closed off by the cervix). To remove them, she just needs to push them out with her PC muscles. She can also jump up and down or just reach inside and pull them out.

Top Three Reasons for Her to Use Ben Wa Balls

1. STRENGTH TRAINING: Using Ben Wa balls helps her strengthen her PC muscles. The benefits of having strong PC muscles are that they provide stronger vaginal grip during intercourse, which feels great for the both of you, and helps her to have more satisfying orgasms. It also helps to prevent problems with urinary incontinence, which means she will be able to withstand your playful tickling for longer without peeing her pants.

2. A SEXY SECRET: She can wear Ben Wa balls all day long. This could make for a fun sexual secret to share as you take her out for a day exploring that beach resort or even doing mundane acts like shopping. Sometimes wearing the balls for several hours can culminate in an orgasm, although this isn't true for everyone. Even if she doesn't orgasm, the secret is mentally stimulating for everyone and can result in extra-hot sex later.

3. NEW SENSATIONS: Speaking of hot sex, she can keep the balls inside while you engage in a little bit of coitus. Men report that the sensation of the smooth balls rubbing against their cock during sex is exotic and feels great. It also gives her that sexy, filled-to-the brim feeling.

BDSM Toys for When She's Naughty (or Nice)

This catchall category includes items such as nipple clamps, restraints, blindfolds, whips, and crops. You don't have to be a dungeon master; BDSM toys can be pleasurable for everyone interested in pushing their sexual boundaries.

Three Exciting Ways to Play with BDSM Toys

1. BLIND PASSION: Add a blindfold to remove her sense of sight so that she won't know what erotic tricks you have in store for her. With her sense of sight missing, her other senses will be heightened. Try playing with her sense of touch by dripping body wax on her skin, tickling her with a feather, or whipping her with a crop. Play with her sense of hearing by snapping a whip in the air to create suspense, or put on some seductive music. Play with her sense of taste Mickey Rourke-style (of *9 1/2 Weeks*) by feeding her a variety of delectable treats, like strawberries, honey, and mango's, and asking her to guess what she's tasting. Play with her sense of smell by lighting aromatic candles or incense sticks.

2. PAIN/PLEASURE: When women are aroused, the line between pain and pleasure can be gloriously blurred. This is why she may like it when you spank her, roughly pinch her nipples, and bite her when she's at the peak of her arousal. Add intensity to this combination by using nipple clamps, whips, and crops. The trick is to reward her pain with a moment of relief, so if you spank her, immediately soothe her bum with a series of sweet kisses or soft stroking. If you clamp her nipples, follow it up with some cunnilingus or kiss her neck.

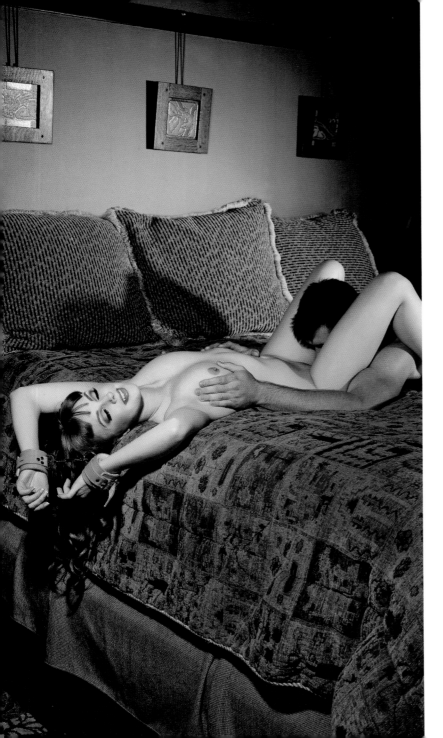

« 3. RESTRAIN HER: There is something extraordinarily tantalizing about being restrained and used for your pleasure. Try a pair of furry handcuffs, scarves, or a set of restraints that restrict both her arms and legs. Tie her up and then tease and tantalize her with your fingers, tongue, cock, and toys. Be sure to only use restraints that she can get herself out of should she need to in case of an emergency. (She might just look so hot tied up that you keel over with a heart attack—you never know!)

Today there are gadgets of all types that enhance every part of our lives, from how we communicate to how we copulate. As a twenty-first-century lover, it behooves you to stock up with a drawerful (or a chestful, or a truckful) of sex toys to help you bring fun, pleasure, and titillating new games to your sex play. And it might just help you help her to that big, toe-curling orgasm she's been craving.

SEXtracurricular Activities: Take Her on a Shopping Date

It's time to stock up your sex toy treasure chest. Take your girl on a shopping date and buy her whatever she wants!

1. MAKE IT A SEXY DATE. Tell your girl that you are going on a naughty, sexy date and ask her to dress up in her favorite skirt sans underpants. (Don't tell her exactly what you're up to, but definitely emphasize that it's *naughty*—you don't want to give her the impression that you're about to take a private jet to Paris or something.)

2. CHOOSE A CLASSY STORE. Visit your nearest female-friendly sex-toy store. (Fascinations, Good Vibrations, and Coco de Mer are a few we love. Do some research to find something similar in your area.) DO NOT, we repeat, *DO NOT* take her to that windowless creepfest porn-and-peep-show shop on the wrong side of town. If you are a particularly shy couple, going online is a good source, but we highly recommend visiting a brick-and-mortar store, as you can actually see and feel the products. Plus, you'll get a little thrill out of the naughty outing.

3. SPOIL HER. Tell your darling that this outing is your treat and that you want her to pick out whatever sexy item her heart, or puss, desires. Women love to be spoiled!

4. TAKE NOTES.
What items does she gravitate toward? Is she lingering in the lingerie section? Does she spend a lot of time investigating the vibes? Is she enticed by the erotica? Or is her interest piqued by porn? This is your chance to learn something about your girl that you might not have known before.

5. HURRY HOME!
It's time to immediately put your new sex toy to the test. Have fun with it and keep adding to your collection. Each time you visit the store, you'll find that both of you are a little more brazen than before.

6. HEED THIS EXPERT NOTE.
If you are purchasing a sex toy as a gift for your partner, Lauren Wolf has the following advice for you: "Choose a product that is quality, classy, nonphallic, perhaps one that is primarily for external use (like the Nea by LELO). You might introduce it for the first time when you are with her, but also be open to giving it to her and allowing her some time without pressuring her to use it right away."

CHAPTER 9

HER BRAIN ON SEX

THE MIND-TO-PUSSY CONNECTION

The biggest sexual organ is the human brain. Without imagination and mental stimulation, we might as well be turtles fucking on the beach. Turtles don't desire romance or sex toys or porn, they don't care about infidelity, and they only know how to do it in one position. (Turtle Style!) What is the connection between the female mind and her pussy? And what does this connection mean to you?

"SEX IS EMOTION
IN MOTION."

– MAE WEST

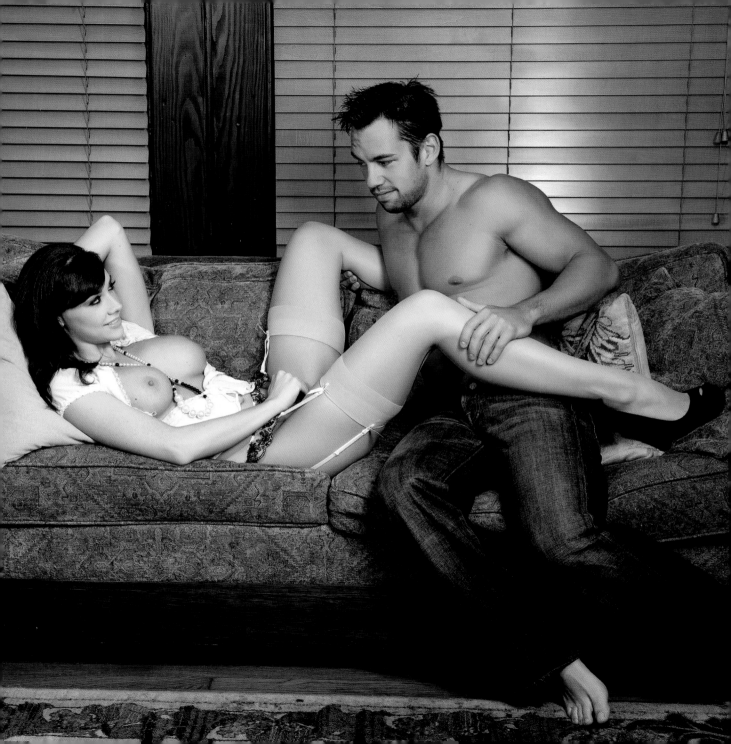

The Heart-to-Pussy Link

Disney taught women to look for Prince Charming—that studly, rich guy from a good family who looks great in tight white pants. (We're talking about Peyton Manning here.) It's Prince Charming (or Peyton Manning) who will show up someday and sweep her off her feet. Beginning with a single kiss, they'll live happily ever after emotionally and presumably sexually.

Even though your average man may not be Prince Charming, if he has a good role model, he has surely been taught the value of emotional intimacy when it comes to dating and getting laid. In our survey, 88 percent of men said that their partner needs to feel an emotional connection to enjoy sex. "It seems to me that a lot of women, mine included, are not physical when it comes to sex. They are more emotional," says fifty-something Wallace. But is this just another stereotype? How closely connected is her heart to her horny bone, anyway?

Which came first, the emotion or the sex? Some scientists postulate that women become emotionally attached *after* experiencing a release of oxytocin brought about by an earth-shaking orgasm. Dr. Ian Kerner says that "during sex, women produce lots of oxytocin, a hormone that stimulates a strong emotional connection. As a result, women are more emotionally integrated when it comes to sex. That's why casual sex and hookups often backfire for lots of women."[44] Says twenty-something Annabeth, "I think sex creates an emotional connection—it's inescapable." Thirty-something Jen tells us, "I don't need to have an emotional connection to jump in bed with a guy. But after sex, the emotional part takes hold, and I'm in trouble." But some women say they won't even copulate with a man unless she feels in some way attached to him. Twenty-something Hannah confesses, "I feel that sex is the ultimate display of emotional, physical, and spiritual connections with a person and should be respected."

And then, of course, there are the women who just love sex, sans the emotional connection. Twenty-something Hayley says, "Some of the best sex I've ever had has been with strangers who just knew exactly what they were doing." And sixty-something Katrina confesses, "I prefer not to have the emotional attachment, it's less complicated."

The lesson? Just like you fellas, women want sex at different times for different reasons. Some women want the whole romantic burrito, others want a nice fat slice (or two) of orgasm pie, while yet others are just looking for a quick-fix hot dog from the street vendor to satisfy their craving. These viewpoints can shift and change as a woman gains new experiences with men. What can we say? Don't pigeonhole your lover, and enjoy the ride.

Masturbation: She Loves to Love Herself

In our survey, we found that a shocking 52 percent of men said they think that women rarely or never masturbate. Boys, boys, boys! What makes you believe this? Do you just go green with envy at the thought of us putting our fingers all over ourselves? Or do you suffer the impression that us gals just aren't into sex unless you are there to convince us that we are? Or perhaps it's the fact that female masturbation is still shaking off its cloak of taboo.

Whatever the reason, we've got some news for you, fellas: Ladies enjoy their solo time and you shouldn't be jealous. In the 2010 *National Survey of Sexual Health and Behavior*, more than half of women ages eighteen to forty-nine reported masturbating during the previous ninety days.[45] And in our own survey of progressive, hot-to-trot chicks, we found that 40 percent said they masturbate a few times per week, and 18 percent said they do so daily.

We hope you are jumping up and down with joy at the news that women enjoy masturbation. Not only is it good for her, it has some darn good repercussions for your sex life, too.

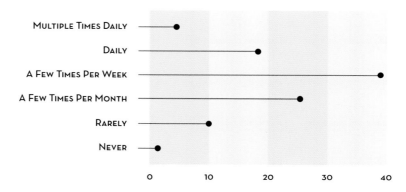

WOMEN: HOW OFTEN DO YOU MASTURBATE?

Forty percent of women said they masturbate a few times per week and only 2 percent said they never do.

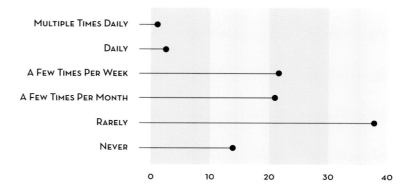

MEN: HOW OFTEN DO YOU THINK YOUR PARTNER MASTURBATES?

Thirty-eight percent of men said they think their partners rarely masturbate, and 14 percent were under the impression that she never puts a finger in her own hooha!

Three Reasons It's Important for Your Girl to Masturbate (and How It Benefits You, Too)

1. EASIER ORGASMS: She needs to know how to achieve an orgasm. If she never touches herself, she'll be hard-pressed to know what works best to get her off. You can benefit from her practicing on herself, as she'll be able to tell (or show) you what types of strokes work best to stoke her fire. It will also make achieving orgasm that much easier for her, alone and in the sack with you. In fact, some sex therapists prescribe daily masturbation for women who have trouble achieving orgasm. Dr. Jenni says, "For a woman to know her body and pleasure, she also needs to know her vulva—as if it's her best friend."

2. SEXUAL CONFIDENCE: A 1990 study by researchers at the University of Utah, Salt Lake, determined that "Women who masturbate appear to hold more positive sexual attitudes and are more likely to be orgasmic than those who don't."[46] A woman who is open to her body's pleasure will be more open to you giving her pleasure. She'll feel sexier, more confident, and more vivacious in bed.

3. STRESS RELEASE: The release of feel-good hormones like oxytocin with orgasm will help lower her stress levels. Women often have difficulty making "me time," but there is nothing more relaxing and mood shifting than giving herself a whopper of an orgasm. It can help her sleep better, too. This will benefit you, since a happy, relaxed woman is a lot more fun to be around.

SEXtracurricular Activities: Put on a Good Show!

Although the majority of the women we surveyed said that they have masturbated in front of their partner, 23 percent of women told us they've never tried it. We think it's time for you two to put on a good show for each other and enjoy a little mutual masturbation.

1. TAKE A SHOWER TOGETHER. Get in the shower and soap her up, massage her shoulders, and play with her nipples or her other hot spots. (Don't touch her pussy though!) Get her relaxed and aroused.

2. TURN THE LIGHTS DOWN LOW. Women are often very shy about showing off their bodies, but it's amazing what dim lighting can do for her confidence. Use a strand of holiday lights, candles, or dimmers.

3. SET THE STAGE. Make the bed and lay out her favorite sex toy (if she has one). Turn on some of her favorite music in the background. Make sure there are no distractions like cell phones or pets. This will help keep her mind engaged as her body lets go.

4. ENCOURAGE HER. Tell her you want to see her touch herself. Be assertive and encouraging when you say this. If she's shy, but willing, persuade her to let go by kissing her neck, stomach, and nipples, and gently taking her hand and leading it to her vulva. Tell her how beautiful she looks and how much you want to see her pleasure herself. (Note: If she's really too shy to relax, don't force her. It's best to gracefully let it go and try again another time.)

5. WAIT UNTIL SHE'S WARMED UP. Once she gets going, take your cock in hand and start masturbating yourself. Continue to tell her how hot she is, how turned on she's made you, and how hard it is to resist taking her.

You may find each other to be too irresistible to finish the job solo, or you might find the game so exciting that you both reach orgasm while watching each other pleasure yourselves. In either case, have fun!

Cheating Chicks

Men aren't the only cheaters; after all, it takes two to tango. Forty-seven percent of our female survey takers admitted to having cheated at least once, and 6 percent said they haven't but that they might someday.

The Top Three Reasons Why Women Cheat

We found three main reasons why a woman might cheat on her man.

1. SEXUAL NEGLECT: A woman who feels consistently sexually unwanted by her partner may be driven to cheat. The only thing that keeps an intimate relationship going is intimacy. Lose this, and one partner is likely to look elsewhere to meet the basic human need of being sexually desired. Says forty-something Lara, "My partner lost complete interest in having sex because he gained a lot of weight. I tried to get him interested in every way I could and eventually went elsewhere because I am a sexual being."

2. PURPOSEFUL RELATIONSHIP SABOTAGE: Sometimes a woman cheats when something else is going wrong in the relationship. Cheating becomes a way of escape or a catalyst for the inevitable break up. Says twenty-something Darian, "I was unhappy in my relationship and had tried to talk to my partner about it. He refused to address the issues and wouldn't acknowledge my feelings. I just got more and more unhappy until I started acting out and cheating—to fulfill emotional needs that weren't being met in my relationship, but also to try to sabotage the relationship."

3. CURIOSITY ABOUT WHAT ELSE IS OUT THERE: Sometimes, when in a long-term relationship, women (and men, too) get curious about what other people might have to offer them in bed. This curiosity could be sparked by a flirtatious coworker or by sudden and intense chemistry with a guy at the bar. Not all women act on these feelings, and many times a woman relegates the curiosity to a fantasy to be savored while masturbating or even while screwing her partner (51 percent of the women we surveyed said they sometimes fantasize about other people while having sex with their partner). But in some cases, curiosity catches the pussy and is enough to lead her to being unfaithful. Says thirty-something Olive, "The first time I cheated was when I was twenty-one. I had gotten married at eighteen and wanted to see if the grass was really greener on the other side. (Not really. It's all just grass.)"

Women and Pornography, Do They Watch the Smutty Stuff?

Hellooo, boys. Have we got news for you! Girls watch video porn too! And it's not necessarily something they only do when having fun with you. The stats from our survey are in, and the results may surprise you. Fifty-four percent of women we surveyed admitted to occasionally watching porn, while a minority of 18 percent said they never watch it. Thirty-six percent of women who do watch porn said they only do so alone and, what's more, 28 percent said their partner doesn't know they visually feast on the dirty smut! Only 9 percent of women said they only watch porn when with their partner. This may explain why 52 percent of the guys we surveyed told us they think their partners never touch the stuff, and 32 percent believed that their girls only look at it when they're chaperoning the fun. Says twenty-something Lynn, "I find porn to be exciting, but also a bit degrading, and for that reason I feel like I shouldn't be aroused by it and have never told a partner that I watch it."

Next time you're at your girlfriend's place, ask her to show you her porn collection—you might be in for a fun surprise.

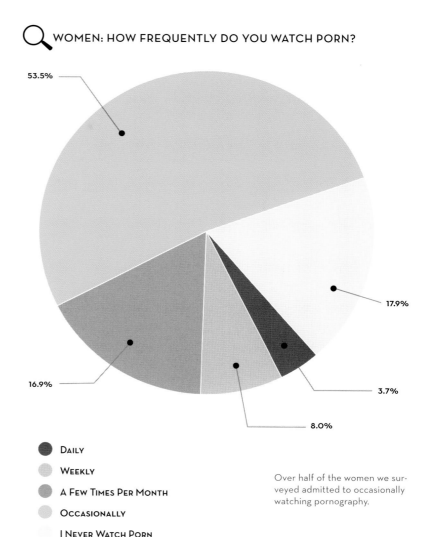

WOMEN: HOW FREQUENTLY DO YOU WATCH PORN?

53.5%

17.9%

16.9%

8.0%

3.7%

- ● Daily
- ● Weekly
- ● A Few Times Per Month
- ● Occasionally
- ● I Never Watch Porn

Over half of the women we surveyed admitted to occasionally watching pornography.

WHEN IT COMES TO PORN, WOMEN ARE PICKY!

Women's views on porn differ from girl to girl. While some enjoy porn for what it is—a fuckfest meant to arouse—others are completely opposed to the stuff.

The majority of the women we talked to enjoy pornography, but they are super-picky about what they will or will not watch. If you're interested in watching porn with your lover, take these things into consideration.

1. IT CAN'T BE DEGRADING. Women aren't saying they don't have an appreciation for rough sex now and again, and there are quite a number of women who enjoy female submission BDSM-fare (where a woman gets tied up and spanked or more). However, there should be no choking, spitting, humiliating, or even facials *unless* it's very clear that the woman on screen is in fact enjoying the treatment. As women, we're very keen to what's going on in that girl's face, it's a part of the feminine brain structure to be more empathetic to other people's emotions than men are,[47] which, paired with our feminist roots, makes us a lot more sensitive to a porn star who is doing a terrible job of acting. If the porn star is not enjoying performing, or if she's being abused, a woman is not going to enjoy watching it.

2. THE ACTORS NEED TO BE ATTRACTIVE. In a lot of porn flicks, a moderately or even very attractive woman is getting heartlessly pounded by a flabby-assed, hairy, big-dicked, headless ape of a man. We feel short-changed when we see videos like this. If sex is going to be filmed, it should be a good show—otherwise, why partake? Says forty-four-year-old Dee, "Usually, porn consists of women you can't identify with being screwed by guys you wouldn't want to touch you. I have never seen a guy in a porn movie who I would want to have sex with." And Lyn, a twenty-something biologist says, "The best porn is the stuff done by natural-looking actors. None of this greased-up, bowling-ball-implant nonsense."

3. IT CAN'T BE BORING. A six-minute Internet clip of a guy jacking off may be just what we're looking for while we're home alone with our vibrator. If we want to be really engaged in the film for any length of quality masturbation or partner sex time, there needs to be substance. This doesn't necessarily mean it has to be of the same cinematic quality of, say, the insanely sexy 1986 movie 9 ½ Weeks (although, wouldn't that be lovely?), but the film needs to have a good balance between sex and plot development.

4. IT CAN'T BE GROSS. Sure, sex is fun when it's dirty. But most girls really aren't going to be thrilled to pieces over a guy hawking a big loogie onto his partner's butthole as lubrication. (There are SO many sexier ways to prepare her for anal sex, guys—and be aware, you shouldn't emulate this move at home with your girlfriend, either.) And we're bound to be distracted by imperfections like pimples on her butt or a scary-looking outie belly button. What can we say? We like things to be classy and well-presented, and that applies to our smut, too.

5. IT NEEDS TO FEEL AUTHENTIC. There should be real chemistry between the actors, and it's thrilling when the woman has an authentic, earth-shaking orgasm (rather than a played-up, fake screamer—and yes, we can tell the difference).

CHEAT SHEET: PORN THAT YOUR LADY MAY LOVE

Here is our suggested porn viewing list for you and your sexy lady to help get you started.

1. Candida Royalle's Femme Productions: Good plots, sexy actors, and hot sex scenes. *www.candidaroyalle.com/*

2. Christina Noir's Wet Box Productions: Run by adult entertainer Christina Noir and her husband. Her movies feature real sex and real people, and they're really hot. *www.wetboxvideo.com/*

3. Tristan Taormino: Her work is about real chemistry and sexy hook-ups. She's also a great resource for sex education. *www.puckerup.com/*

4. Maria Beatty and Bleu Productions: For something a little edgier, this is a collection of lesbian BDSM and fetish porn movies. *www.bleuproductionsonline.com/*

PRESCRIPTION: MORE PORN

The doctor is in, and she's telling you that porn can be good for your sex life. So long as you are both up for it and you've selected fare that the two of you can enjoy together, pornography can be a great way to add a little fun to your bedroom shenanigans.

Here are the top three reasons why porn can be good for your sex life.

1. MOVIES CAN BRING IN NEW AND FUN IDEAS TO TRY. Sometimes when you've been in a relationship for a while, the sex can get pretty rote. Download a porn flick and you both might discover some new and exciting positions, locations, or role-playing scenarios to try.

2. IT CAN HELP YOU COMMUNICATE YOUR DESIRES MORE EASILY. Have you always wanted to try anal sex, fisting, or a little bondage? Put on a film that reflects your fantasies and see how your partner reacts. This saves you the trouble of having to articulate some of these pervy thoughts aloud, but still opens up the door to let your wild side shine through.

3. PORN CAN ADD SOME NAUGHTY FANTASIES WITHOUT RUINING YOUR RELATIONSHIP. Although an orgy or a threesome may sound fun and exciting to the both of you, sometimes the reality of a fantasy come true is a little too much to handle (jealousy, STDs—you know, that kind of stuff). Turn on a porn flick that features what you both have been dreaming of and live out your fantasy in your minds while you play together in safety.

OTHER STUFF TO STIMULATE HER SENSES

Video porn is only a small part of what's available to you and your partner to enhance your sex lives (and it may not even be high up on her list of turn-ons). Other stimulants like sex toys (read Chapter 8), erotica, role playing, and dirty talk will help round out your sexual relationship.

A clit-ologist should include the following in his bedroom arsenal.

1. EROTICA: In our survey, 72 percent of women told us that they enjoy reading written erotica as a prelude to masturbation. Use this to your advantage. Stock up on a few sexy reads or visit some of the many sexy websites out there dedicated to erotic short stories. Find a story that you like, perhaps one that reminds you of her or something you'd like to do with her, and offer to read her a bedtime story. The sexy story will undoubtedly inspire her to enjoy a little storytelling of her own.

2. THINGS TO STIMULATE HER IMAGINATION: Titillate her mind before you titillate what's between her thighs. Try a game of sexual role playing. She could be your naughty student and you a reprimanding teacher. Or you could play the part of the fix-it guy who has come to fix her leaky pipes. Sure, you two may laugh, but if you can get beyond the initial silly feeling, you might find that you are really on to something.

3. DIRTY TALK: A lot of women enjoy the art of dirty talk. If you aren't well versed in giving great lip service, it's probably best to start slow and work your way from mild to on fire. Whatever you do, don't progress from one level to the next if you can tell she's just not feeling your adjectives, verbs, and nouns. Here are some ideas to get you started:

- Mild: "You look irresistible in that dress; it makes me think things that I really shouldn't be thinking."
- Medium: "I hope you're not wearing panties, because I might just have to tear them right off of you."
- Hot: "I'm going to bend you over the counter and give you a spanking so I can see my handprints on your ass."
- On Fire: "You've been a naughty little slut, haven't you? I'm going to have to fuck you so hard that you won't be able to see straight."

Once you've become an eloquent smut-talker, try kicking it up a notch by telling her a dirty story while you're having sex. Use your imagination and spare no detail.

Cheat Sheet: Erotica Reading List

Here are our top picks to start your erotica collection.

1. Look for anthologies edited by Rachel Kramer Bussel, Kristina Wright, Jordan LaRousse, and Samantha Sade (yes, that's us!), Maxim Jakubowski, and Violet Blue.

2. If you're looking for some BDSM reading, try the Sleeping Beauty series by Anne Rice or the classic *The Story of O* by Pauline Reage.

3. Want a little romance? Try authors Opal Carew, Kresley Cole, Colette Gale, and C.J. Barry.

4. Exciting erotica websites include OystersandChocolate.com, Literotica.com, and CleanSheets.com.

Now *That's* Kinky!

We asked men whether their partner has ever expressed interest in any kinky activities. The survey results show that more women are interested in BDSM and swinging than their men might have known about. Seventy percent of the women we surveyed told us that they're open with their man about what they want in bed. But what about the other 30 percent? Are they just shy?

"I WOULD LIKE TO FUCK A GUY WHILE WEARING A STRAP-ON DILDO."

—KITTY, 27, TEACHER

WOMEN: ARE YOU INTERESTED IN THE FOLLOWING FETISHES/SEXUAL PREDILECTIONS?

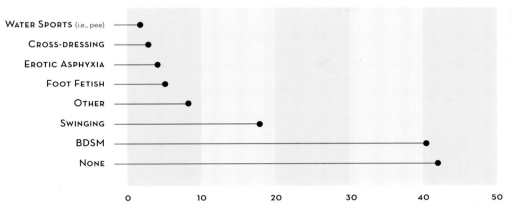

Forty percent of the women we surveyed reported having an interest in BDSM, while 19 percent reported an interest in swinging.

MEN: HAS YOUR PARTNER EXPRESSED INTEREST IN THE FOLLOWING FETISHES/SEXUAL PREDILECTIONS?

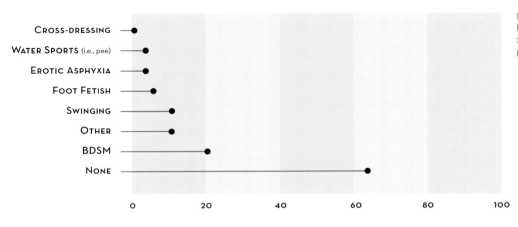

Men seemed to underestimate how kinky women can be. Only 22 percent suspected their partner might be into BDSM.

LURE YOUR KINKSTRESS INTO THE OPEN

What should you do if your girl is on the shy side? Here are two games your woman is sure to enjoy that will allow her to open up about the sexy things she'd like to try in a way that is fun and feels safe.

1. THE ALWAYS, SOMETIMES, NEVER LIST: Relationship coach Elaina McMillan (www.bringbackthatspark.com) recommends the Always, Sometimes, Never List to help a couple learn about each other's fantasies. You can either write out the list or just tell each other your thoughts while you are cozied up under the covers. First, tell each other what you are ALWAYS up for in the sack. This could include things like oral sex and massages. Then list the things that you are SOMETIMES up for. Everyone's list will be different, but hers may include things like sex in dangerous locations, giving a striptease, or making a homemade porn movie. Then you tell each other what's on your NEVER list. Some people might include things like threesomes or going to strip clubs, while others may have broader boundaries and only include acts that are illegal or nonconsensual on this list. Whatever the case, you'll certainly have the opportunity to learn a lot about each other and hopefully open the conversation to try something new and exciting.

2. THREE FANTASIES IN A HAT: Each of you write down three fantasies, each on a separate piece of paper, and toss those papers into a hat. Be honest and write down something that you've really wanted to try but just haven't had the courage to bring up. This could be as innocent as waking up to hot morning sex or something as daring as trying anal sex for the first time. Then pull a fantasy and decide whether or not you want to try it together. The key here is that you need to approach each other's fantasies without judgment. If you pull a fantasy that you are absolutely not willing to try, let her know that it sounds hot but you're just not comfortable with it and move on to the next one. Hopefully, you'll discover that you've both been aching to try out some of the same things.

Gentlemen, don't make the mistake of thinking that your lady is a "good girl." Many women are a lot naughtier than they let on, but are often afraid to express their desires for fear of being labeled a slut or not worthy of a romantic relationship. If you want to keep your lady happy and sexually satisfied, it's important to open up the doorway to her fantasy world. Don't be afraid to find out what she really wants in her dirtiest of dirty desires—and if it's exciting to you, by all means, give the girl what she wants!

CHEAT SHEET: DIRTY GIRLS!
WOMEN DISH THEIR NUMBER ONE FANTASIES

"To be in an X-rated theater having sex or masturbating
with my man while others watch."
—*Jade, 57, communicatress*

"To have sex outside, under a blanket of stars."
—*Stephanie, 21, nanny*

"Being with an older more experienced man who takes advantage of me."
—*Samantha, 26, accountant*

"Being with a man that enjoys oral sex—giving and receiving."
—*Noel, 56, project manager*

"To be on a tiny deserted island with a lagoon, cabana, and hammock.
Lounging, sunning, and having sex all over the place."
—*Nalani, 48, massage therapist*

"To be a sex slave, tied up, used, spanked, taken by stranger after stranger
while my master facilitates the whole experience."
—*Mimi, 32, ob-gyn*

"Watching another lady jerk off my husband."
—*Girly, 54, banker*

"I would love to be a woman in the middle of enjoying four guys.
One on each boob, sucking my nipples, one eating me out, and me sucking the other
one off. And they're all under the age of thirty-five! Pure cougar fantasy!"
—*Dee, 44, real estate agent*

HAVE YOU TRIED, OR WOULD YOU EVER TRY, ANY OF THE FOLLOWING KINKY ACTIVITIES?

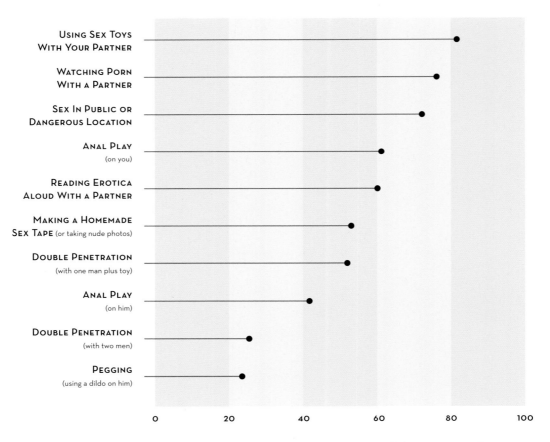

Eighty-two percent of women we surveyed use, or want to use, sex toys. The least popular activity was pegging, but it still accounts for nearly a quarter of our ladies being up for it!

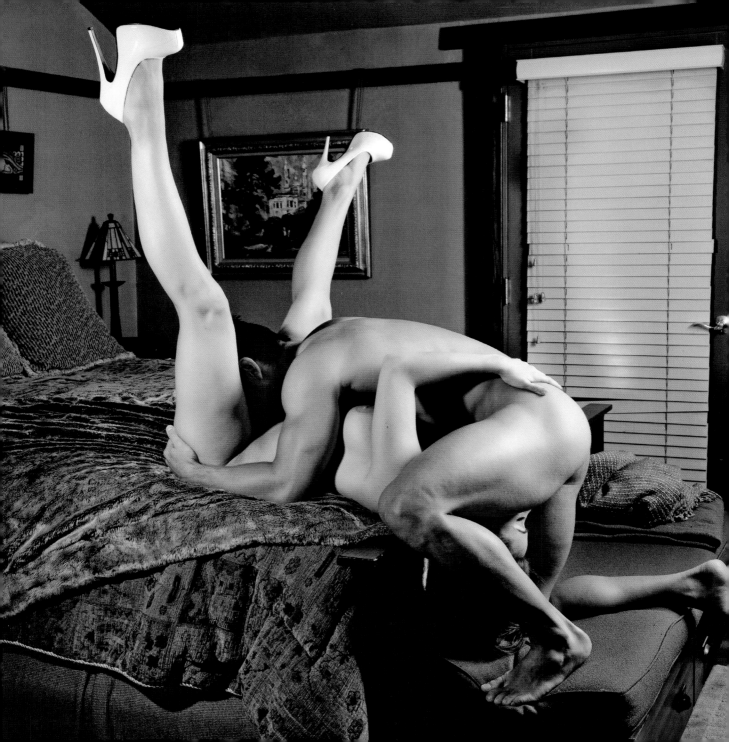

CHAPTER 10

HER LIBIDO

FROM WILD GIRL TO COLD SHOULDER, WHAT DOES IT ALL MEAN?

For many men, a woman's libido, otherwise known as her sex drive or desire, is a thing of mystery. Popular culture would have us believe that a man's sex drive is a constant, reliable thing, kind of like a loyal dog, always on and always ready to play. On the flip side of the same token, a woman's sex drive is often painted as never matching a man's, finicky, hard to understand, up and down, on and off, and wily—something that's hard to pinpoint and often rife with contradiction, perhaps more like a kitty cat. However, all of this is not always as simple (or as boring) as some would have us believe. The sex drive and sex function of both men and women are complex animals. Let's explore her libido, the ins and outs of what affects it, and how you can help stoke it from an ember to a raging fire.

"SEX PLEASURE IN WOMEN IS A KIND OF MAGIC SPELL; IT DEMANDS COMPLETE ABANDON; IF WORDS OR MOVEMENTS OPPOSE THE MAGIC OF CARESSES, THE SPELL IS BROKEN."

– SIMONE DE BEAUVOIR

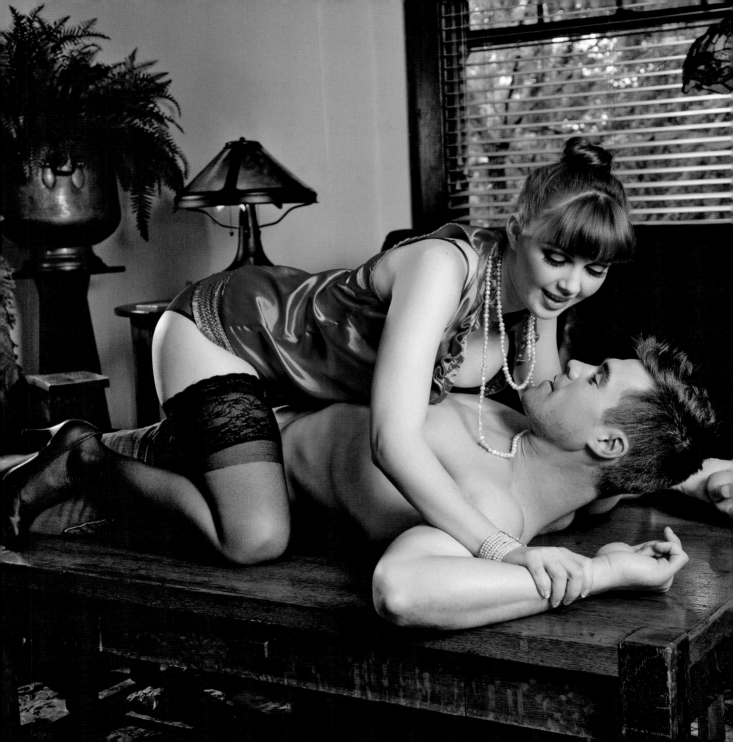

CHEAT SHEET: WHAT WOMEN SAY MOST ATTRACTS THEM TO A MAN

"His ambition and drive."
Michele, 46, greenhouse grower

"His honesty and openness."
—Linda, 48, mom

"His voice! I'm a sucker for a guy with a nice speaking voice."
—Chanti, 40, nurse

"If he looks at me like something desirable, I'm likely to respond!"
—Shelly, 39, educator

Other qualities that received several honorable mentions include your teeth, your hands, and your confidence.

SHE WANTS SEX MORE THAN YOU THINK SHE DOES

It is often argued that men think about sex more often than women and want it more often than their female partners. There are certainly social factors out there that support these notions, such as the existence of so many strip clubs geared toward straight men and the huge pool of mainstream pornography created for men. Much of this is the result of the social constructs that shape gender attitudes and expectations about sex. We want to help you to see your lover's libido in a different light and give you the necessary information you need to embrace, nurture, and play with it to create the very best sex life you both can have.

In the OystersandChocolate.com surveys, we asked both men and women separately how often they wanted to be having sex. The results showed that the desire of men and women are surprisingly close!

The lesson here? Perhaps she wants sex more often than you think she does! Or perhaps (since we can assume that most of the women we surveyed are erotica readers because they found the survey through our erotic website) you ought to find a lover who likes reading smut! Either way, these numbers indicate that the sex drives of men and women may be more evenly matched than we're all lead to believe.

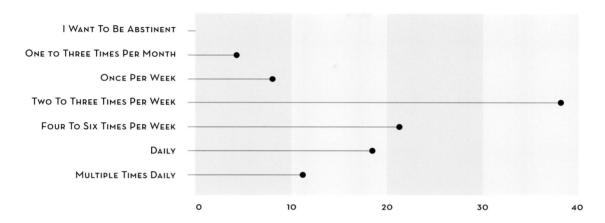

MEN: HOW FREQUENTLY DO YOU WANT TO BE HAVING SEX?

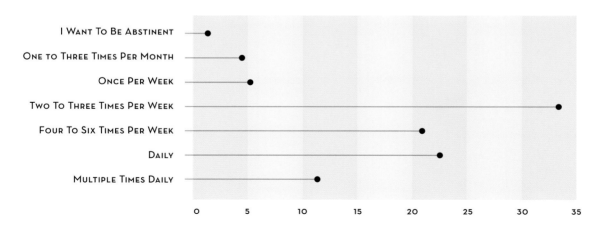

WOMEN: HOW FREQUENTLY DO YOU WANT TO BE HAVING SEX?

Love Her Libido

Rather than thinking of your lovely lady lover as having a weaker libido and inferior interest in sex in general, we'd like to encourage you to think of her as having a fluid, flavored, and multifaceted libido. It's a beautiful thing, always in flux, and because it can be stoked by so many different stimulants, that just makes it all the more fun for you! You may just find that joining her on an adventure into the land of her sexual desire can be thrilling and full of sexy surprises that you might have been overlooking.

Let's look at a few of the factors that influence her libido and discuss how you can engage them to keep her excited about sex with you.

A Is for Attraction

The first and most basic ingredient in the alphabet soup of desire is her attraction to you. For some women, it's that first glimpse of you from across the room—the way you carry yourself and the sparkle in your baby blues (or big browns, or gorgeous greens)—that gets her heart a-racing. For other women, it's after she's gotten to know you a bit and finds your sense of humor and intelligence absolutely panty-wetting. The important thing for you is to find out what she is attracted to and nurture it.

The take-home for you is that, for women, what's inside really does count and can make up for any physical attributes you may be lacking.

B Is for Boredom

Nothing is going to kill her libido like boredom, fellas. Sometimes, even if you have her coming on cue during your very regular and scripted sex routine, the boredom factor will still dampen her desire. Try to mix it up a little. You can always fall back on those tried-and-true techniques once it's time to get her off. Here are some ideas to get those creative juices flowing.

1. Surprise her with a new sex toy, and use it.

2. Each sex session, pick a different body part to concentrate on and spend a minimum of five minutes licking, kissing, and nuzzling said body part. (Read Chapter 7 for ideas.)

WOMEN: WHAT FEATURES ARE IMPORTANT TO YOUR SEXUAL ATTRACTION TOWARD A MAN?

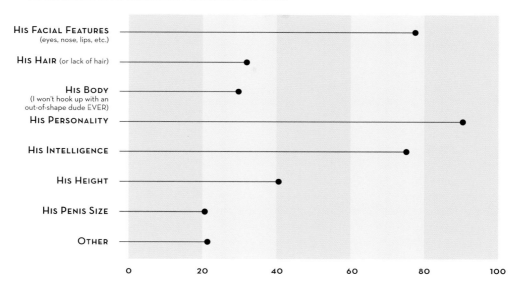

His Facial Features (eyes, nose, lips, etc.)

His Hair (or lack of hair)

His Body (I won't hook up with an out-of-shape dude EVER)

His Personality

His Intelligence

His Height

His Penis Size

Other

0   20   40   60   80   100

The women we surveyed told us that your personality (91 percent) and intelligence (76 percent) rank as some of the most important features when it comes to sexual attraction.

3. Look at the positions in Chapter 5 and try a different one for each sex session. When you run out of new positions, check out the *Kama Sutra* and try some of those moves.

4. Have sex in the car. Or outside on the lawn furniture. Or on your mom's couch.

5. Talk dirty and make noise. Many women love aural stimulation almost as much as oral stimulation.

C Is for Chemistry

Chemistry between the two of you will go far in feeding her desire. Does she love the way you smell without any cologne or other products on? This is a good indicator that there is a natural chemistry there. It turns out that there is an evolutionary basis for why smell is so important when it comes to sex. Researchers from the University of Bern in Switzerland did a smell test on a group of women, having them smell an assortment of T-shirts, each of which had been worn by a different man for two nights. The women were asked to rate the man's body odor, pleasantness, and sexiness. It turns out that women much prefer scents exuded by men whose genetic immune system profiles (more precisely, histocompatability complexes—MHC—a collection of genes that are related to the immune system) vary the most from their own, which would in turn mean that they would have healthier offspring. The women unknowingly smelled and rejected shirts that were worn by men with similar MHC complexes to their own, and many went as far as to say it reminded them of a brother or a father's smell.[48] What this means for you is that some women will be naturally attracted to your scent (most likely, those with dissimilar immune systems), and some will not.

While you can't do anything to affect the natural chemistry you two share, you at least now know that if she truly loves your man musk, she'll be more interested in having sex with you on a basic, animalistic level. You can use this to your advantage by hopping into bed with her right after your shower but before you cover up that sexy man-essence with deodorant, aftershave, or cologne.

L Is for Lusty Lifestyle

Exercise and healthy eating are key to keeping your lover's libido in tip-top shape. When she eats well and exercises, she'll look and feel more beautiful, which typically translates to her feeling sexier and more sensual as well. Twenty-something Vanessa tells us, "I keep active and healthy so I have the desire and physical capability to enjoy sex with my boyfriend, who also does the same. Keeping myself in shape makes me feel sexy, which boosts my confidence and makes sex more enjoyable, both for me and my partner."

Aerobic exercise, such as running and brisk walking, increases heart rate, improves blood flow, and releases endorphins into the body (which cause an overall feeling of well-being). Deep stretching, such as yoga, increases blood flow to the pelvic area and improves circulation to her genitals, which will improve her sexual arousal and orgasmic function. Strength training helps her body produce more testosterone, which is an important element in her feeling horny.

Exercise also helps fight stress and fatigue, which are major libido killers for women,[49] and it always helps with her body image—another important element that, when healthy, keeps her libido fit as well.

Eating right falls along the same lines as exercise. Eating a diet high in "bad" fats, like those found in processed foods and fast food, and foods high in sugar will make her sluggish and add on the pounds, both of which are bad for her self-image and energy in the bedroom. If she's eating a balanced diet full of "good" fats—such as those is found in nuts, fish like salmon, and avocados—as well as plenty of fruits, veggies, and whole grains, she'll be well-fueled for some sensational time spent in the bedroom. We recommend you promote a healthy diet for her by participating in it with her. Eating well together means fucking well together.

P Is for Any Physiological and Psychological Factors

Here is a list of physiological factors, such as specific medications, that can affect her sex drive, which she probably should talk to a doctor about.

THE BIRTH CONTROL PILL: The pill works by tricking her body into thinking it is pregnant. The hormones in the pill have been shown to decrease libido in women because their bodies don't naturally produce as much androgen or testosterone, hormones that are important to sexual arousal.

Contraindication Warning

Guys, if you value your sex life and sanity, don't ever, *EVER* approach your lover and tell her she needs to hit the gym. You telling her she needs exercise will produce an adverse reaction, side effects of which might include, but are not limited to: a) you sleeping on the couch, b) a drastic decrease in blow jobs, c) cold dinners, and d) lots of tears and nasty looks, which will necessitate a huge amount of cuddling with no sex involved.

If you feel like a little physical activity might be good for your sweetie, suggest something that the both of you can do together, and word it in such a way that indicates you're just doing it for the joy of it or that you personally feel you could use a bit of exercise and need her help to stay inspired. A few ideas include rollerblading, hiking, swimming, or playing basketball together.

SEXtracurricular Activities: Feed Her Lust

Aphrodisiacs are foods (or other substances) that stimulate sexual desire. And for women, there's nothing sexier than a man cooking in the kitchen. Surprise her with a romantic evening and a meal. Can't boil water without burning it? Present her with a platter of ready-made morsels. Either way, she'll appreciate the thought, romance, and effort—all of which will keep her sexual desire healthy and burning. Here are a few aphrodisiac foods to incorporate into your presentation.

1. CHOCOLATE: It may seem cliché, but quality chocolate contains PEA (phenylethylamine), often called the love chemical. PEA naturally occurs in the brain and is in particularly high levels when a person falls in love, inducing feelings of euphoria and excitement.[50] Serve her chocolate truffles or chocolate-covered strawberries.

2. HOT PEPPERS: If your lover likes it a little spicy, make her favorite Mexican dish with some hot peppers thrown in. Hot peppers contain capsaicin, which increases heart rate, rate of breath, sweating, and blood flow—all reactions when a person becomes sexually excited, as well.[51]

3. OYSTERS: Yes, some say they resemble female genitalia. But they are also high in zinc and have been linked to increased testosterone production—a necessary hormone for your lady love's libido.[52]

Other foods that have historically been considered aphrodisiacs include basil, strawberries, honey, artichokes, rosemary, coffee, asparagus, grapes, and avocado. While there is little scientific backing behind the idea that these foods truly make her horny, all are delicious and sensuous to eat—reason enough to serve them up for your libidinous meal.

DEPRESSION: True depression is a physical and mental problem that makes a person feel sad, listless, angry, drowsy, upset, and more. As many as 75 percent of people with depression report a loss of sex drive. Unfortunately, many medications used to treat depression also cause a drop in sexual interest. It's important for a woman to discuss both depression and medications in terms of her sexual drive with her doctor to find what will work best for her.

HISTORY OF SEXUAL ABUSE: Sexual abuse can affect a person at so many different levels. If your lover has a history of abuse, it's important that she seek medical and psychological help.

HER MONTHLY CYCLE

We asked the men we surveyed what they noticed about their lover's monthly hormonal cycles, and how those cycles affected their sex lives. The range of answers we received was amusingly broad. Joe, a forty-one-year-old computer programmer, told us, "I've noticed that my wife gives off a pheromone the week before her period, and it drives me crazy with desire." Jon, IT project manager, age thirty seven, wondered, "Wow, am I really this oblivious?" And Benjamin, a twenty-eight-year-old novelist, replied, "She never uploaded the schedule on my planner. I wasn't aware there was going to be a test on it."

CYCLE BASICS

As G.I. Joe reminds us, "...knowing is half the battle." The more you know about your lover and her body, the better lover you'll be. For all of the Jons and Benjamins out there, let's go over the basics of her cycle, shall we?

Most women experience a twenty-eight-day cycle, which kicks off during puberty. In broad terms, the cycle begins when the brain releases chemical messengers and hormones, which trigger a few of her eggs to mature and one to release. Your lover will ovulate fourteen to sixteen days before her period, and if your sexy sperm don't fertilize the egg, she'll begin her menstrual flow, which usually lasts four to eight days.[54]

VALERIE WANTS VIAGRA

The little blue pill has done much for men and their sex lives, and it has many people curious about what it could do for the fairer sex. Sildenafil, the active drug in Viagra, basically works by increasing blood flow to the penis. But what about the clitoris? H. George Nurnberg, M.D., of the University of New Mexico School of Medicine in Albuquerque, led a four-year study between 2003 and 2007 that observed the effects of sildenafil on women who were taking SRI antidepressants, such as Zoloft, Prozac, and Paxil, which have been known to negatively affect sexual function. The women chosen for the study had reported a variety of sexual problems, including trouble becoming lubricated, delay in achieving orgasms, and/or lack of achieving orgasm at all. The researchers found that 72 percent of the women on Viagra were "much improved" or "very much improved" on a scale of sexual functioning, compared to 27 percent of women on a placebo who reported the same result.[53]

The FDA hasn't approved Viagra for women, but doctors sometimes prescribe it off-label in certain cases when a woman's sexual function is affected by her antidepressant. They do not, however, prescribe it to increase sexual desire or drive.

What Her Cycle Means for You

Following is a basic guide as to what you might encounter over the course of a woman's cycle. Remember that every woman is different, and not all follow a twenty-eight-day pattern—their cycles can be longer or shorter. You may want to observe your lover and learn what specifically happens with her from week to week; all the better to know when it would be best to plan to spend the weekend cleaning out the garage, or when to plan a romantic massage date for the two of you.

WEEK 1: (beginning the first day after her period is over): Her energy levels are higher than during her period and, for many women, her mood is lighter. You may notice her coochie will produce less natural vaginal lubrication during sex. (Time to stock up on Astroglide!)

WEEK 2: Her body is approaching ovulation. Her cervical secretions are wetter and more slippery and may be whiter than at other times of the month. As she approaches the end of the second week, she will most likely start to ovulate. Some women may experience breast tenderness, a few mood swings, and an increase in libido.

WEEK 3: Her vaginal secretions may dry up a bit, and her mood may balance out.

WEEK 4: She'll experience premenstrual symptoms, and then her period. These can include mood swings, bloating, cramps, insomnia and/or fatigue, cravings for specific foods, and digestive issues.[55]

A Note on PMS and Diet

There is new information out there that a lot of premenstrual syndrome (PMS) is caused by poor diet or vitamin deficiencies. PMS does run in the family, but other things can compound it or make it worse, such as when she doesn't get enough vitamin B6, calcium, and/or magnesium. Too much caffeine can also make it worse, as well as high levels of stress and lack of physical activity.[56] Many of the guidelines for a healthy lifestyle we discussed earlier will help with her PMS symptoms. Throw in a multivitamin, and some TLC, and the two of you should do just fine.

Hysterectomy: What Does It Mean for Your Sex Life?

A hysterectomy is a procedure wherein a woman's uterus is surgically removed. Also, with some hysterectomies, the ovaries may be removed (an oophorectomy).[57]

If you are with a woman who is going to have or has had a hysterectomy, there is a special set of sexual circumstances you should be aware of.

If your lover's ovaries are not removed, her body should still produce the female hormones necessary for a healthy sexual drive. However, going through a surgery that removes part or all of her uterus can affect her body and mind in other ways. After going through the proper recovery time, some women feel an increase in libido because they no longer have to worry about birth control or getting pregnant. They may also feel an increase in libido if they had a lot of bleeding and pain before their surgery that is now no longer present.

Other women may experience a decrease in sex drive because they enjoyed the feeling of uterine contractions against their cervix during orgasm (which will no longer occur). Some may experience great sadness at the loss of the opportunity to have children, or any more children, as the case may be. And still other women may be psychologically affected by the simple knowledge that her uterus is gone. Unfortunately, health experts still don't fully understand the physical and psychological affects that hysterectomy has on women.[58]

If your lover has her ovaries removed, there will most definitely be a hormonal effect on her sex drive. It will be similar to what she might go through during and after menopause, and is sometimes referred to as surgical menopause. She will experience a cessation of her period, hot flashes, night sweats, mood swings, sleeplessness, fatigue, and/or anxiety. There are a variety of hormone replacement therapies she can look into. She should work with her doctor to find what's best for her body.

It's important that you communicate openly with your lover and support her in getting any medical attention and/or therapy that she feels she needs. And of course, do everything you can to make her feel loved and sexy!

Advice from the Front Lines: How Best to Deal with a Lover's Mood Swings

Here's some advice our male survey respondents had to give about how they handle their lovers when experiencing bad mood swings.

- "Just be a loving partner and don't take things to heart...it's not different than someone having a bad day."

- "Leave town! Actually, just be as patient as possible, don't try to fix anything."

- "Be gentle and understanding."

- "Find a project or household chore to do, and shut up. Let it roll on past."

- "Stay away and say the word 'YES' a lot."

- "Talk about it. A woman's period is a natural part of life and if partners talk about it, it saves a lot of headaches and hurt feelings."

- "Haul ass if necessary. Assume sainthood otherwise."

- "ooh FUCKING HELL..."

- "Well, there's mutually assured destruction, I suppose. It's how we handled the Cold War, and that worked out fine. Sort of."

THE MYSTERIES OF MENOPAUSE

Menopause is an important, transformative event in a woman's sexual and hormonal life, and with it comes changes to your sex lives. Know that for many couples, sex after menopause is adventurous and amazing.

The number of a woman's eggs decreases throughout her life and becomes very low when she enters into her mid- to late forties. Her ovaries then begin to fail to release eggs, which in turn affects the amounts of estrogen and progesterone that the ovaries produce. Menopause actually refers to the last period a woman will have, which can happen anywhere between ages forty and sixty, with the most common age being fifty-one. However, the process of her reproductive system slowing down, referred to as perimenopause, involves the three to five years before she stops menstruating, during which her body will go through many changes and her periods will become irregular.[59]

The Change, as it's so eloquently called, will have an emotional and physical affect on your lover, the extent of which varies from woman to woman. Of the women we surveyed, 28 percent said their sex drives remained the same over the course of menopause as they had been before the Change, and that number rose to 47 percent for postmenopausal women. Even better, 33 percent said their sex drives increased during menopause and postmenopause.

Because of her lower estrogen levels, the biggest sexual changes she will most likely encounter will be vaginal dryness and thinner vaginal walls (which might make her more tender during sex). Your lover and her doctor may decide that hormone replacement therapy (HRT) is a good choice for her, which may counteract the dryness and thinning. But for you personally, your best friend to deal with these two conditions is LUBE!

Now that you are educated on the various factors that influence your partner's libido, you can approach her sexuality with a bit more understanding. While her sex drive may be susceptible to a great number of influences, such as her attraction to you in particular and her body's wily hormones, it's best for you not to underestimate her libido. Beneath most women's calm and cool exterior is a flame just waiting to be properly stoked and lit to a raging, sexy inferno. Once you get her started, we wish you the best of luck in keeping up with her.

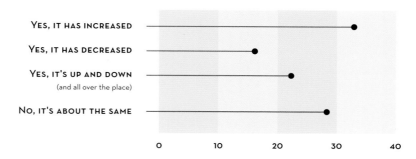

IF YOU'RE GOING THROUGH MENOPAUSE, HAS YOUR SEX DRIVE CHANGED?

Yes, it has increased

Yes, it has decreased

Yes, it's up and down
(and all over the place)

No, it's about the same

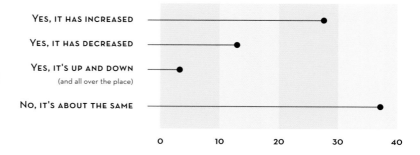

IF YOU'RE POST-MENOPAUSAL, HAS YOUR SEX DRIVE CHANGED?

Yes, it has increased

Yes, it has decreased

Yes, it's up and down
(and all over the place)

No, it's about the same

CHAPTER 11

Big-Bellied Mamas

Pregnancy and Childbirth and Its Effect on Her Sexuality

With all of the sex practice you're hopefully getting (especially after you finish reading this book and become a bona fide clit-ologist), some of you may actually get around to making a baby or two. Forty-two percent of men we surveyed think sex with a pregnant partner is really sexy! Says Alex, a forty-something attorney, "It's hot knowing she's growing your baby inside her. Physically, her skin is clearer, her breasts are bigger, her pussy is hotter, tighter, and wetter... What's not to like?" Having a pregnant lover is a special, wacky adventure, because a woman's body and hormones change in ways that are unique and specific to those forty weeks. Let's go over some of the things you may encounter in a pregnant lover, as well as tips on how to navigate those big-bellied months for some sexy, preggo fun.

ALISON SCOTT:
"I'M PREGNANT."
BEN STONE:
"PREGNANT...
WITH EMOTION?"
ALISON SCOTT:
"PREGNANT WITH
A BABY."

- KNOCKED UP (2007)

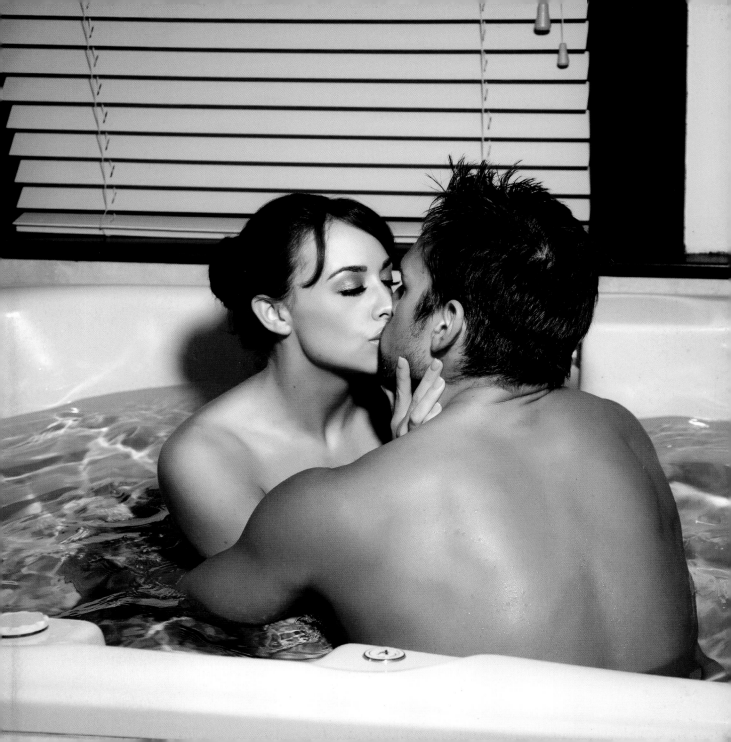

What to Expect from Her Hooha When She's Expecting

Your female lover's body will go through tremendous hormonal and physiological changes over the duration of her pregnancy. While her mood and state of horniness can and most likely will change from day to day, and even from moment to moment, many women have some consistent experiences throughout each of the trimesters.

A Titillating Full Term

1. SEX IS A-OKAY. Sex between monogamous, committed, healthy partners is considered safe at any stage of a normal, low-risk pregnancy. The notion that sex is dangerous during a normal pregnancy is now an antiquated one. Follow your doctor's or midwife's instructions.

2. TREAD LIGHTLY. Be aware that your lover will be very different than when she's not preggo, hormonally speaking. This means that she may be far more emotionally sensitive than usual. A little joke or lighthearted tease that used to make her laugh might now inspire water works. Save the sarcasm for boy's night out, at least for these nine months.

3. SHE RUNS HOT AND COLD. You may feel like your partner's sex drive is a moving target. Says Mumette, 33, a stay-at-home-mom, "My sex drive seemed to fluctuate. I didn't want to be touched at all during the first trimester, my second trimester was full of awesome orgasms but no sex drive, and my third trimester was my horniest." Shelly, a thirty-something writer, reports, "Oh God, my sex drive goes way up when I'm pregnant—I'm a lot hornier and less inhibited, too. Everything is more sensitive. Until the last two or three weeks when I'm actually very horny but the belly and everything else just makes it too difficult." Be understanding of her changes and just go with the flow.

Her First Trimester

1. Now that neither one of you have to worry about her getting knocked up, you may find you both feel more relaxed and have an increased desire for sex. Enjoy!

2. With the upsurge of hormones, your partner may have an increased sex drive that will continue through the three trimesters.

3. Her breasts will swell to prepare to produce milk for the little bambino, and they'll also become more sensitive—if she was the kind of girl who loved it rough, she may prefer soft touches and gentle licking instead.

4. Most women experience nausea and fatigue during the first trimester. Now is the time to spoil her with foot rubs and gentle cuddles. "Feeling sick is not a gateway to sexiness," comments thirty-something Lily.

5. Her orgasms may feel more intense or lingering. Some women will love this, but it might be uncomfortable for others. Pay attention and ask questions as you help her navigate these new sensations. Says forty-something L.L., mother of four, "During my pregnancies, sex is always as good as the best sex when I am not pregnant."

Her Second Trimester

1. Her nausea and fatigue will most likely start to lessen in the second trimester, which means (hopefully) she'll have more interest in sex!

2. She will most likely begin to show—some women respond to this by feeling feminine and sexy while others may feel fat or unattractive. Try to be sensitive to how she's feeling and shower her with compliments and praise. Says New York City Midwife Jocelyn Hart, "Sex can be more interesting during the second trimester. Her vagina gets bigger with increased blood flow, and there are more vaginal secretions. Her breasts will be larger, and, of course, her belly is swelling. These physical changes can be very exciting."

Knock, Knock

Some men are afraid that they will hurt the baby if they have intercourse with their pregnant partners. If you're one of these guys who worries that your dick is going to knock the poor little one around and give him or her brain damage, let us assure you that the baby is quite safe. Baby is protected by the strong muscles of the uterus as well as the amniotic sac. There's also a mucus plug that seals her cervix,[60] so your penis cannot possibly come into contact with the fetus during intercourse.

Contraindication Warning

Doctors don't warn against oral sex during pregnancy, but there is a danger if you blow air into her vagina, especially during the third trimester. If you blow into her vaginal opening and the cervix is slightly open, air bubbles can enter into the blood stream and cause an embolism. This can be fatal to her! So if you go down on her, DO NOT huff and puff into her hole.[62] This is also a risk postpartum—especially when her vagina is still healing if she had a vaginal birth. Whatever you do, stick to licking; no blowing, Moby Dick!

3. Mid-pregnancy, your lover may start secreting colostrum from her nipples. It's "a yellow or clear, thick, sticky substance that is the baby's first food," says Hart. "It's high in protein and immunoglobulin."

4. You may start to feel some of the baby's movements, especially toward the end of the second trimester. Don't worry, you're not going to hurt baby, and he or she has no idea what's going on when you two go at it.

5. As her pregnancy advances, there is increased blood flow to the entire pelvic area, which means her vulva and vagina will be more engorged. This typically equates to more pleasurable orgasms, and even multiple orgasms. Many women claim that the best sex of their lives occurs during the second trimester of their pregnancy. Moreover, because of the increased blood flow to the vulva and vagina, her vagina may feel tighter to you[61] (a sensation that most men enjoy)—so gentlemen, take advantage of her swollen, sexy state!

6. Increasing estrogen levels mean increased vaginal secretions.[63] If she was one who usually needed to use lube, you'll now have the pleasure of getting to splash around in her natural, sweet juices instead!

Her Third Trimester

1. Your lover's belly will truly blossom during the third trimester, and her breasts will continue to swell. Says Joel, a thirty-something business manager about his pregnant partner, "Her body is changing, her breasts are getting bigger, and she's just beautiful." However these big changes can equate to some real discomfort on her part, so now, more than ever, is the time to be loving, playful, and creative when it comes to sex!

2. As she gets closer to her due date, her orgasms may inspire mild contractions in her uterus. These are called Braxton Hicks contractions and are nothing to worry about (unless she is at risk for preterm labor or her doctor has other concerns).

3. Be aware that because of the engorgement of her vulva and vagina, she may seem to be sexually insatiable. Many women express that even right after an orgasm, they still feel unbelievably horny. On the flip side, some women experience this as extreme discomfort and may not want any sex at all.

4. The cervix is ripening in preparation for eventual labor, so if your cock is big enough to hit her cervix, there may be some spotting. This is normal and no cause for concern, but if it makes you both feel better, try some sexual positions that encourage shallower penetration, such as Spoons. In this position, the woman lies on her side with her legs closed, and you "spoon" up behind her. Her closed legs will keep the penetration mellow, and the snuggle factor in this position is a bonus. Positions that have her on top are also great, such as the traditional Cowgirl position, wherein you lie on your back and she kneels over you. These positions allow her to control the depth of penetration. An added bonus is that you can help do some of the heavy lifting by grasping her ass from below if she gets tired. (Read Chapter 5 for more shallow-penetration moves.)

> "SEMEN CONTAINS A SUBSTANCE CALLED PROSTAGLANDIN THAT CAN HELP 'RIPEN' THE CERVIX, WHICH MEANS IT CAN HELP THE CERVIX SOFTEN AND EFFACE (THIN OUT). THIS HELPS THE WOMAN GO INTO LABOR IF HER BODY IS READY TO DO SO, BUT IT DOESN'T ACTUALLY INDUCE LABOR."
>
> —JOCELYN HART, MIDWIFE

SEXtracurricular Activities: Lubin' Her Up and Rubbin' Her Down

Massage and touch are especially important when it comes to a healthy sex life with your knocked-up partner. Rubbing her the right way will not only help relax her and ease some of the more painful parts of pregnancy, but it may just get her in the mood, too!

1. Use a high-quality brand of cocoa butter to rub her belly, lower back, hips, and bottom. The cocoa butter will help soothe the pull of her skin over the growing baby, and will also help prevent pesky stretch marks.

2. Use a light-scented lotion that contains vitamin E to rub her breasts and nipples. Both become engorged during pregnancy, and her nipples can become irritated, stretched, and dry, as well.

3. Gently massage her perineum. Some experts believe that keeping her perineum well-lubricated, especially right before delivery, will help prevent vaginal tearing during birth. (And even if it doesn't, the touch will feel amazing.) Use a water-based lubricant (e.g., K-Y Jelly), olive oil, vegetable oil, or vitamin E oil.[64] This can also be a great addition to your oral sex sessions.

Expert Tip: Pillow Magic

Cunnilingus is one of those fabulous sex moves that should fit the bill throughout all of her stages of pregnancy. If she's uncomfortable on her back, or if her doctor has recommended she stay off of it, Ian Kerner, Ph.D., recommends placing a pillow underneath her hip and lower back and tilting her slightly to either side.[65]

Cheat Sheet: Positions and Techniques for Fun Playtime with Your Pregnant Lover

Keep in mind that your lover is pregnant, not sick or fragile. In general, make sure that you both are comfortable and that you don't put your full weight (or your lover's) on her pregnant belly or too much pressure on her uterus. The following are suggestions for some hot preggo lovin'!

1. It's your lucky day, boys. The overwhelmingly recommended best position from pregnant women is Doggy Style. It's not rocket science to figure out why this might be so: Your sexy preggo lady on all fours with you saddled up behind and inside her gives her ample space for her belly (at any stage of pregnancy). Nice variations include her on the bed and you kneeling behind her, or her on the bed, but close to the edge, and you standing behind her. Do be careful, especially toward the end of her term, that you don't penetrate too deeply if her cervix is sensitive, because this position allows for some incredible penetrative depth.

2. Standing Doggy Style is another position to try. Your partner stands and leans forward either on the bed, a chair, a table, or the back of the couch (whichever is most comfortable for her height). This position allows her to rest on whatever piece of furniture she's leaning on, while you stand behind her and go to town.

3. In Side to Side, you both lie on your sides facing each other, she lifts one leg over your hip, and you enter her. This position works for most couples until the end of the term because you can angle her to accommodate her belly, and it's also nice if you're craving the intimacy of Missionary, but she can't lie on her back.

No Sex or Orgasms Equals No Fun for a While

Some women will have certain risk factors during pregnancy that may cause her doctor to advise she not have penetration of any kind (i.e., with fingers, toys, or penises). This is the perfect time to tune in and tone up on your clitoral techniques (for tips, read Chapters 1 and 3). If she can't even enjoy orgasms, but she loves giving head or hand jobs, you may weather the no sex/no orgasm storm just fine. However, chances are, her discomfort will have her feeling less than giving. Reserve this time for kissing and hugging and holding hands, and feel free to take lots of long, solo showers.

Postpartum Sex: Getting Busy After She Delivers

Some men (and women) see sex as a big question mark after the baby is born. There will definitely be a period of time during which your lover will be healing and won't be able to have penetration. There will also most likely be a longer period of time during which the two of you will be exhausted and just won't be in the mood for sex of any kind. The important things to remember are to follow the doctor or midwife's instructions and to be patient with one another. Don't have sex until you're given the go-ahead, and don't have sex until you both feel completely comfortable with it and you both want it. "There is no magic date, and really no science to the six-week rule or postpartum appointment to have sex. I always counsel 'There is no specific time; when you feel ready and it doesn't hurt, it's okay to go ahead,'" advises Hart.

Treat Her to Some Lube

After a hundredfold increase of estrogen levels during pregnancy, your lover's estrogen levels will drop after birth. This will lead to vaginal dryness—so, lube her up!

Breastfeeding: Mix Her Milk With Her Cocoa Puffs

Hormonal changes found in breastfeeders are said to result in a lower desire for sex. These changes include a drop in estrogen (a female sex hormone), a drop in androgen levels (sexual desire hormones), and an increase in prolactin (a hormone that

Fact or Fiction: Her Vagina Will Be Looser and Won't "Feel as Good"

A common concern after childbirth is that a woman's vagina will never be quite the same—that it won't be as tight or toned. While it's true that your lover's vagina goes through quite a stretch to pass that baby, know that the female form is an amazing thing. It may take a year or longer, but if she does her Kegel exercises regularly, her vagina will return to its prebirth, tip-top, toned, snug fit (if she never did Kegels before, she may have even more sexy muscular control now). Read Chapter 5 for the proper technique for Kegel exercises. It's a good idea to do them at a regular time every day, such as during baby's first morning feeding.

decreases sexual desire). However, sex pioneers Masters and Johnson found that breastfeeders have an increased desire for sex when compared to their nonbreastfeeding counterparts. How could this be? One theory is that the hormonal changes brought on by breastfeeding are often offset by sex itself, an activity which increases oxytocin and dopamine levels—hormones that accentuate feelings of desire and love.[66] So what does this all mean? Basically, breastfeeding is a natural act and so is sex. You, as a couple, can partake in both. Just be aware that when you lick her nipples, her breast milk is not going to taste like your basic 2 percent cow's milk; it has a sweeter, heavier taste and texture. Cream, anyone?

Set the Stage

Here are a few more things you can do, to ensure that sex picks up and continues at some point.

- If you can afford it, hire a house cleaner. The fewer household chores and responsibilities the both of you have to worry about, the more attention you can give not only to your baby, but also to the intimacies of your own relationship.

- Make out, if only for a minute or two. When she's throwing impossibly tiny socks into the dryer, come up behind her, wrap your arms around her, turn her around and kiss her, for at least forty-five seconds. Even though it may not lead to a full-on, passionate romp session in the laundry room, gestures such as these will remind you both how fun it was to get into this baby mess in the first place.

- Set a date night every week. The romance in your partnership needs time to flourish without the needy little one around every second of every day.

A pregnant woman as a lover and a partner is unlike anything else. We hope you experience it as the opportunity it is, not only to grow together intimately, but to have some out-of-this-world, shoot-her-to-the-moon-and-beyond, wild, crazy, loving sex that's only possible with your pregnant lady.

1. Strong, Bryan. *Human Sexuality: Diversity in Contemporary America*. New York: McGraw Hill, 2008. Print. p. 70.

2. "Designer Laser Vaginoplasty Toronto | DLV." *Toronto Cosmetic Surgery Clinic—Breast Augmentation and Liposuction Specialists*. 2006–2011. Web. 11 Jan. 2011. www.tcclinic.com/designer-laser-vaginoplasty.php.

3. Chalker, Rebecca. *The Clitoral Truth: The Secret World at Your Fingertips*. New York: Seven Stories, 2002. Print. pp. 11–12, 35.

4. Ford, Paul. "Take the Downtown Train." *The Morning News*. 25 May 2004. Web. 11 Jan. 2011. www.themorningnews.org/archives/personalities/take_the_downtown_train.php.

5. Strong, p. 76.

6. Chalker, p. 43.

7. Chalker, p. 47.

8. Chalker, p. 50.

9. Leigh, Jasmine. "Faking It—Ask Men." *AskMen—Men's Online Magazine*. ING Entertainment. Web. 03 Jan. 2011. http://www.askmen.com/dating/vanessa_150/152b_love_secrets.html.

10. Winks, Cathy, and Anne Semans. *The New Good Vibrations Guide to Sex*. Pittsburgh, PA: Cleis, 1997. Print. p. 103.

11. Masters, William H., and Virginia E. Johnson. *Human Sexual Response*. Toronto: Bantam, 1981. Print.

12. Masters and Johnson, p. 128.

13. Kerner, Ian. "Give Her Multiple Orgasms—AskMen.com." *AskMen—Men's Online Magazine*. 2009. Web. 02 Feb. 2011. www.askmen.com/dating/love_tip_300/384c_love_tip.html.

14. Koedt, Anne. "The Myth of the Vaginal Orgasm by Anne Koedt." University of Illinois at Chicago website. 1970. Web. 02 Feb. 2011.www.uic.edu/orgs/cwluherstory/CWLUArchive/vaginalmyth.html.

15. Ellis, Albert, and Shawn Blau. *The Albert Ellis Reader: A Guide to Well-being Using Rational Emotive Behavior Therapy*. New York: Citadel, 2000. Print. p. 14.

16. Masters and Johnson, p. 59.

17. Masters and Johnson, p. 67.

18. "Sex Trivia—Interesting Sexual Facts about Both Animals and Humans—The Sex EZine." The Lilith Gallery of Toronto. Web. 14 Jan. 2011. www.lilithgallery.com/articles/sex/Sex-Trivia.html.

19. Kerner, p. 55.

20. Winks and Semans, p. 17.

21. Kerner, p. 55.

22. Hite, Shere. *The Hite Report: A Nationwide Study of Female Sexuality*. New York: Seven Stories, 2004. Print. p. 285.

23. Zdrok, Dr. Victoria. "Mastering A Woman's G-spot—AskMen.com." *AskMen—Men's Online Magazine*. Web. 18 Jan. 2011. www.askmen.com/dating/vanessa_100/115b_love_secrets.html.

24. Donaldson James, Susan. "Sex Study Says Female Orgasm Eludes Majority of Women—ABC News." ABCNews.com. 4 Sept. 2009. Web. 20 Jan. 2011. http://abcnews.go.com/Health/ReproductiveHealth/sex-study-female-orgasm-eludes-majority-women/story?id=8485289.

25. Angier, Natalie. *Woman: An Intimate Geography*. New York: Anchor, 2000. Print. p. 71.

26. Joannides, Paul. *Guide to Getting It On!* Waldport, OR: Goofy Foot, 2006. Print. p. 267.

27. "Anatomy—The Healthy Prostate.com." The Healthy Prostate.com—Home. Web. 17 Jan. 2011. www.thehealthyprostate.com/anatomy.html.

28. Winks and Semans, p. 15.

29. Winks and Semans, p. 134.

30. "Anal Sex Safety and Health Concerns." WebMD—Better Information, Better Health. Ed. Louise Chang, MD. 17 Nov. 2010. Web. 17 Jan. 2011. www.webmd.com/sex/anal-sex-health-concerns.

31. Winks and Semans, p. 130.

32. Winks and Semans, p. 131.

33. "Anal Sex Safety and Health Concerns." WebMD. 17 Nov. 2010. Web. 17 Jan. 2011.

34. Winks and Semans, p. 73.

35. Joannides, p. 287.

36. "Anal Sex Safety and Health Concerns." WebMD. 17 Nov. 2010. Web. 17 Jan. 2011.

37. Henley, Jon. "America Reveals Its Sexual Secrets | Life and Style | The Guardian." The Guardian, Guardian.co.uk. 5 Oct. 2010. Web. 08 Feb. 2011. www.guardian.co.uk/lifeandstyle/2010/oct/05/sex-us-american-attitudes-survey.

38. Joannides, p. 280.

39. Berman, Dr., Laura. "The Science of Sex Appeal." Oprah.com. Harpo Inc., 03 Apr. 2009. Web. 25 Jan. 2010. www.oprah.com/relationships/The-Science-of-Sex-Appeal/2.

40. Strovny, David. "Erogenous Spots—AskMen.com." AskMen—Men's Online Magazine. Web. 12 Dec. 2010. www.askmen.com/dating/love_tip/32_love_tip.html.

41. Fox, Kate. "The Smell Report—Sex Differences." Social Issues Research Centre. Web. 24 Jan. 2011. www.sirc.org/publik/smell_diffs.html.

42. Maines, Rachel. The Technology of Orgasm: "Hysteria," the Vibrator, and Women's Sexual Satisfaction. Baltimore, MD: Johns Hopkins UP, 1998. Print. p. 135.

43. Margolis, Jonathan. O: the Intimate History of the Orgasm. New York: Grove, 2004. Print. p. 191.

44. Kerner, Ian, and Tracey Cox. "The Biggest Sex Mistakes Men and Women Make—Relationships." TODAYshow.com. 27 Sept. 2007. Web. 08 Feb. 2011. http://today.msnbc.msn.com/id/20955254/ns/today-relationships/.

45. "The Kinsey Institute—Sexuality Information Links—FAQ." The Kinsey Institute for Research in Sex, Gender, and Reproduction. 2010. Web. 08 Feb. 2011. www.kinseyinstitute.org/resources/FAQ.html#masturbation.

46. Strong, p. 281.

47. Eliot, Lise. "Girl Brain, Boy Brain?" Scientific American. 08 Sept. 2009. Web. 08 Feb. 2011. http://www.scientificamerican.com/article.cfm?id=girl-brain-boy-brain.

48. Furlow, F. Bryant. "The Smell of Love: Why Do Some People Smell Better to You? A Look at How Human Body Odor Influences Sexual Attraction." Psychology Today (2008). Web. 27 Jan. 2010. www.pascack.k12.nj.us/70271921145153/.../The_smell_of_love.pd.

49. Varekamp, Nancy. "Can Exercise Boost Your Libido?" Livestrong.com—Lose Weight & Get Fit with Diet, Nutrition & Fitness Tools. Lance Armstrong Foundation, 28 Sept. 2010. Web. 30 Jan. 2011. www.livestrong.com/article/252028-can-exercise-boost-your-libido/.

50. "Psychoactive Food," Chocolate: Directory of Chocolatiers. Web. 31 Jan. 2011. www.chocolate.org/.

51. Shulman, Matthew. "The Science of Aphrodisiacs—U.S. News and World Report." Health News Articles—U.S. News Health. 19 Aug. 2008. Web. 29 Jan. 2011. http://health.usnews.com/health-news/family-health/sexual-and-reproductive-health/articles/2008/08/19/the-science-of-aphrodisiacs.

52. Edmonds, Molly. "The Science of Aphrodisiacs: Science of Love: Science Channel." Science Channel. Web. 29 Jan. 2011. http://science.discovery.com/holidays/valentines-day/aphrodisiacs/aphrodisiacs.html.

53. Nurnberg, George H.; Paula L. Hensley; Julia R. Heiman; Harry A Croft; Charles Debattista; Susan Paine. "Sildenafil Treatment of Women with Antidepressant-associated Sexual Dysfunction: A Randomized Controlled Trial." *JAMA* 2008;300(4):395–404.

54. "Menstrual Cycles: What Really Happens in Those 28 Days?!" Women's Health Information: Feminist Women's Health Center in Washington State Provides Abortion, Birth Control, Reproductive Health Care at Cedar River Clinics. Website Addresses Birth Control, Abortion, Feminism, Pro-choice, Menopause, Contraception, Breast Health, Menstruation, Fertility Awareness, Family Planning, HIV, Emergency Contraception. Web. 28 Jan. 2011. www.fwhc.org/health/moon.htm.

55. "Female Fertility Signals of Ovulation." Menstruation, Fertility, Infertility, Charting Cycles, Conception, Contraception and Women's Health. Web. 29 Jan. 2011. www.menstruation.com.au/fertility/fertilitysignals.html.

56. "PMS (Premenstrual Syndrome): Causes, Symptoms, Diagnosis, and Treatment." Women's Health Center: Information on Women's Wellness, Nutrition, Fitness, Intimate Questions, and Weight Loss. 19 June 2008. Web. 25 Feb. 2011. http://women.webmd.com/pms/premenstrual-syndrome-pms-topic-overview.

57. "Hysterectomy." Women's Health Center: Information on Women's Wellness, Nutrition, Fitness, Intimate Questions, and Weight Loss. Ed. Mikio A. Nihira, MD. 15 Jan. 2010. Web. 01 Feb. 2011. http://women.webmd.com/hysterectomy-8/types-of-hysterectomy.

58. "Hysterectomy." New York State Department of Health. Jan. 2010. Web. 01 Feb. 2011. www.health.ny.gov/community/adults/women/hysterectomy/.

59. "Menopause: What to Expect When Your Body Is Changing." Familydoctor.org. Aug. 2010. Web. 01 Feb. 2011. http://familydoctor.org/online/famdocen/home/women/reproductive/menopause/125.html.

60. "Sex During Pregnancy." KidsHealth, Nemours Foundation. Web. 13 Jan. 2011. http://kidshealth.org/parent/pregnancy_center/your_pregnancy/sex_pregnancy.html#.

61. Sears, Bill and Martha. "Enjoying Sex While Pregnant." Dr. Sears Official Website: Parenting Advice, Parenting Books & More. 2006. Web. 13 Jan. 2011. http://www.askdrsears.com/html/1/T011308.asp.

62. Samuels, Mike, and Nancy Samuels. *The New Well Pregnancy Book.* New York: Simon & Schuster, 1996. p. 116. PDF

63. Sears, Bill and Martha. "Enjoying Sex While Pregnant." Web. 13 Jan. 2011. www.askdrsears.com/html/1/T011308.asp.

64. Pregnancy.org Staff. "Perineal Massage." Pregnancy.org. Web. 13 Jan. 2011. www.pregnancy.org/article/perineal-massage.

65. Kerner, Ian. p. 217.

66. Davis, Elizabeth. *Women's Sexual Passages: Finding Pleasure and Intimacy at Every Stage of Life.* Alameda: Hunger House, 2000. p. 124. PDF.

ACKNOWLEDGMENTS

The most surprising thing about writing this book was learning how much prejudice and misinformation have influenced "scientific" understanding of female sexuality over the years— and how politicized it has all been.

We'd first like to acknowledge the pioneers who have come before us, who have championed women's sexuality and who have worked hard to break down the walls of assumption and inaccurate beliefs when it comes to our bodies. These include, but are not limited to: William Masters and Virginia Johnson; The Federation of Feminist Women's Health Centers; Rebecca Chalker; Mae West; Boston Women's Health Book Collective; Margaret Sanger; Cathy Winks and Anne Semans; Gloria Steinem; Ian Kerner; and Tristan Taormino.

Our utmost gratitude goes to the awesome experts interviewed for and quoted in this book (our personal heroes): Jocelyn Hart, Lauren Wolf, and Jenni Skyler.

Many thanks go to our female friends, both online and in the flesh, who've shared their intimate experiences and dirty details about sex with us so that we could write a more comprehensive, honest book.

Much appreciation to Jill Alexander and the team at Quiver.

And last but not least, much love goes to any man who has the desire and takes the initiative to learn about women's bodies and become a better lover.

ABOUT THE AUTHORS

Jordan LaRousse and Samantha Sade are the authors of *Penis Genius* and *Mastering Your Man from Head to Head* and are the co-owners and co-editors of the premier online magazine for women's erotica, Oysters & Chocolate (www.oystersandchocolate.com). The site is home to the popular sex-advice Q&A column "Ask Jordan," numerous erotic toy, video, website, and product reviews, and the wildly popular weekly sex-tips email. Through Oysters & Chocolate, the duo strives to not only provide quality literary erotica, but to engage women from all walks of life in the topic of sex in a fun and informative way.